FAITH MILLER, D.C.

THE REAL REASON *YOUR* BACK *(still)* HURTS

Discover *Bad Back Syndrome* And What *You* Can Do About It

Published by Performance Publishing, Charleston, South Carolina.
An imprint of Advantage Media.

Performance Publishing is a registered trademark, and the Performance Publishing colophon is a trademark of Advantage Media.

Printed in the United States of America.

10 9 8 7 6 5 4 3 2 1

ISBN: 978-1-961781-84-9 (Paperback)

Layout design by John Hirayama.

Performance Publishing is an imprint of Advantage Media Group. Advantage Media helps busy entrepreneurs, CEOs, and leaders write and publish a book to grow their business and become the authority in their field. Performance Publishing authors comprise a community of industry professionals, idea-makers, and thought leaders. For more information, go to performancepublishinggroup.com.

DISCLAIMER

The information contained in this book is ONLY intended to provide helpful and informative material on the subject addressed. Neither the publisher nor the author expects this book to serve as professional medical advice or replacement for consulting a qualified health professional regarding the reader's specific situation and/or condition. The author and publisher expressly disclaim all liability for loss or damage allegedly arising directly or indirectly from the use or application of any procedure and/or guidance offered in this book.

Table of Contents

Part 3: Take Your Bad Back and Make It a Good Back

Part 4: Keep Up to Join Up

Acknowledgements

This book reveals *Bad Back Syndrome* as the REAL cause of back pain and problems. It's a condition that NOBODY's heard of, EVERYBODY's got, and sadly, FEW know how to handle. *Bad Back Syndrome* is the condition this self-guided manual intends to define and remedy by bringing forth new concepts and a new method that WILL challenge old thoughts and systems.

First, I must give credit where it is due. The information found within these pages was inspired by the CBP® Technique and the late Dr. Donald D. Harrison, who dedicated his life to establishing the principles and procedures practitioners like myself have relied on for reversing mechanically-based backbone problems. This book is rooted in that sound science. With deep respect for his work, I present my version, a simplified method for taking a Bad Back and making it a Good Back.

What you are about to learn regarding *Bad Back Syndrome* is long overdue. Nevertheless, with the arrival of this publication, the general public can finally *understand*, and practitioners can finally *recognize* that back problems are NOT mysterious, and NOT complicated. With *The Bad Back To Good Back Method*, **anyone** can **restore** their problematic back.

This book has been a labor of love, condensing years of tried-and-true testing from patients who undoubtedly had patience with me, applied the method, and made their Bad Back good again. Thank you all for helping me develop this system. I am also grateful to our photo models, my good friend Celene for her tireless editing and enthusiasm, and my husband John, for years of trust and support.

Foreword

It was summer, and I was out on the lake with our three boys. I bent over the side of the boat to pull a ski out of the water, felt something 'give' in my back, and quickly realized I couldn't lift my upper body to get back into the boat. My wife was on shore and ran to the end of the dock when she saw me sprawled out on the back seat. How they got me off the boat and into her office, I haven't a clue. It's all fairly blurry right now, but one thing is entirely clear: she didn't panic.

Things finally calmed down after she worked on me for a few days, and that's when I began to appreciate what my wife did for her patients. Until then, I had no idea. I mean, I supported her through her education and years of clinical practice. She took care of my back occasionally, but then again, I didn't have a need. As far as I was concerned, everybody else needed her more than me. Looking back, now that I've had first-hand experience, I can tell you she didn't panic because she didn't care!

She didn't care that I couldn't stand up straight or walk very far, very fast, because the pain was so bad; she said it would subside. She didn't care that I couldn't get dressed or sit at my desk; she said everything would return in time. Her name is Faith, and with good reason, I trusted her to fix my back so I could get back on my feet, but that's not what she did. She doesn't believe in "patching up" the problem. "Patching up" what problem? I asked her. That was the day I finally understood what my wife's work was all about. It was through her answer to my question that I learned what she really cared about.

She cares about the bones and only the bones. That's why she didn't give a hoot about the agony I was in every time I turned my body or the shooting pain down my leg. She said it wasn't my discs, nerves, or muscles that caused my injury. What happened to me, as I've come to understand, was the fault of my bones and where they ***were*** *compared to where they* ***should have been****. She said THAT was the problem. I didn't know I had a problem because I didn't have any pain or other indications until that day.*

With Faith's guidance, I took my bad back and made it good. She taught me how, and I've continued to keep it good on my own, so I don't have to rely on her. I now know she does care, but maybe that's not quite right either; she loves to help people make their bad back good again.

When Faith and I moved back home several years ago, she told me she wanted to retire from clinical practice and write a book. I cannot tell you how excited I was to learn that, and that is why I've eagerly helped her achieve her goal. She is a fantastic coach and extremely passionate about helping people learn how to take care of their own back.

John Miller

Introduction

Years ago, I began listening to patients describe their back pain. They'd point to where it hurt, try to remember how long it had been burning, stabbing, achy, dull, or radiating, then twist or bend to prove those movements aggravated their condition. Some complained that their debilitating neck and shoulder pain developed into a headache and caused them to miss work, while others grumbled that their nagging low-back issues made it challenging to golf or get out of bed. Most just wanted to know, *"What's WRONG with my back, and why does it STILL hurt?"*

Many patients had tried natural therapies and exercise to relieve their symptoms because they were told their problem was joint or muscle-related. If their nerve or disc symptoms were severe, they'd use medications and receive injections, but the majority bounced from practitioner to practitioner before finding me. Faced with a frustrated patient, I would say, *"I understand how you feel, but you haven't been addressing the right problem."*

Word spread quickly that I was different from other practitioners, and people started showing up at my office because I explained their condition in ways they had never heard before. Sure, I investigated complaints and neurological involvement with physical exams and imaging studies, just like all the others. However, unlike them, I didn't blame a patient's back problems on pain, muscles in spasm, or arthritic joints that were **stuck**. I didn't blame pinched nerves, ruptured discs, or metabolic disorders like obesity, bowel, or thyroid dysfunction. Instead, I blamed a patient's back problems on the REAL problem... *Bad Back Syndrome.*

Isn't My Back Problem Real

You may wonder, *"Isn't my bulging disc, nerve compression, sciatica, headache, or arthritis a real problem?"* Yes, these are real, but they are the result of *Bad Back Syndrome*. Allow me to clarify:

Bulging Discs (C5-C6, C6-C7) that were caused by a head-on collision you had several years ago have left your arms riddled with pain and symptoms that haven't improved. The recommendation was to undergo surgery to cut away the discs that had squished out from between your neck bones. This may sound logical because surgery takes away the damaged tissue and snips nerves, so you can't sense the pain—but *Bad Back Syndrome* remains.

Low Back Nerve Compression caused a sharp, stabbing pain in your back as you bent down to pick something up off the floor. Suddenly, your knees gave out, down to the floor you went, and there you lay for a good while because you couldn't move in any direction without experiencing that same knife-like stab. You were rushed to the emergency room, given meds, and sent home to let the inflammation subside because that's all they found to be the problem. But weeks later, you have just as much discomfort. *What's going on? Bad Back Syndrome* causes nerves to inflame, muscles to spasm, and after they finally *calm down*, the "syndrome" is still around.

Sciatica causes an annoying, burning pain that travels down your butt into your leg. It happens every time you drive. You can't blame a *bulging disc* or *compressed nerves*, but you can blame *Bad Back Syndrome* because it stretches, strains, and aggravates the crap out of the sciatic nerve.

Tension Headaches have caused you to suffer for more than a decade despite medication and routine massages. You remain convinced the painful, sometimes debilitating tension at the back of your head is linked to your stressful job. While stress can compound any type of *headache*, blame *Bad Back Syndrome* for muscle tension.

Arthritis in your lower back (L4, L5, S1) makes it challenging to sleep, and every morning, you wake up with an achy and stiff back. *Why are* *your joints degenerated in ONLY that area and not throughout your entire back? Bad Back Syndrome* is the reason.

What I'm trying to say is that *Bad Back Syndrome* comes first. Your current back problem and any other muscle, nerve, joint, or disc condition occurred secondary to *Bad Back Syndrome.* It's why you've tried every pill, potion, product, procedure, and practitioner, and it's why you continue to complain that your back hurts. If you were addressing the REAL problem, *Bad Back Syndrome,* you wouldn't STILL be suffering from the same or worse complaints.

I've Never Heard Of Bad Back Syndrome

You may question that *Bad Back Syndrome* is the source of your pain and suffering, primarily because you've never heard the term. You are correct. Nobody's heard of *Bad Back Syndrome* until now. Still, I can assure you it's responsible for your neck, middle-Back, and low-back complaints, in addition to problems you would **never... even... consider** being caused by the "syndrome," like *plantar fasciitis.*

I point out *plantar fasciitis* because many of our patients had to end their trail-running days due to the annoying, sharp pain that traveled from their calf muscle down to the heel of their foot. In Step 3, I explain why *plantar fasciitis* is *Bad Back Syndrome's* fault, and throughout the book, it gets blamed for other conditions because it's at the root of ALL problems. Every problem needs a solution, and as you are about to discover, the solution to *Bad Back Syndrome* is that it **CAN... BE... REVERSED**!

First, read all about the "syndrome" so you can know for yourself why it's the source of your back problems. Next, discover your *Bad Back Syndrome Type,* your REAL problem, so you will know exactly what's wrong with your back. Then, use *The Bad Back To Good Back Method* to make your Bad Back good, and lastly, join *The Good Back Club.* This incredibly easy-to-follow, results-oriented guide is designed for anybody ready to DITCH their back problems permanently.

The Good Back Club Starts Here

This is the club you will want to be part of, and when you finally get to join, it will be because you no longer have the "signs" of a Bad Back, but more importantly, you'll be able to PROVE you have a Good Back. This is your journey:

Step 1: Get To Know The Good Back

Step 2: Find Out What Makes The Good Back Go Bad

Step 3: Learn And Observe The Obvious Bad Back Signs

Step 4: Learn And Observe The Not-So-Obvious Bad Back Signs

Step 5: Discover The Bad Back Types

Step 6: Determine Your Bad Back Type And *Quirky's*

Step 7: Master The Methods To Restore Your Good Back

Step 8: Follow The Good Back Rules

Step 9: Apply The Good Back Habits

Step 10: Prove Your Bad Back Is A Good Back

Taking your Bad Back and making it a Good Back won't happen overnight, but AFTER you implement *The Bad Back To Good Back Method,* it could happen in 12 months. Some things just CAN'T be rushed. Countless people have been helped with this system, and it can help you, too. Say **goodbye** to your long-standing back problems, and get ready to join *The Good Back Club*!

Part I

WHY YOUR BACK HURTS

STEP 1: GET TO KNOW THE GOOD BACK

This step is the best place to start your journey, especially if you believe your back pain and problems are a mystery or that they are SO complicated; neither is true. The back is a system of parts. When its parts are strong, stable, and springy, the back is good. If you can grasp how a Good Back **functions** (this step), it will be easier to understand how it **malfunctions** and becomes a Bad Back (Step 2).

GOOD BACK BASICS

The back is made up of 33 bones that descend from smallest (neck) to largest (sacrum). These bones are organized into 4 parts: neck (cervical), middle-back (thoracic), low-back (lumbar), and sacrum (sacral base and coccyx). Each part is sized appropriately for the "load" (body weight) they must carry. Of the 33 bones, only 24 are moveable (7 neck, 12 middle-back, and 5 low-back). The 9 bones comprising the sacrum and coccyx are semi-fused and fused, so they don't really move. Discs are wedged between 23 of the 24 movable bones. There is NO disc between neck bones #1 and #2.

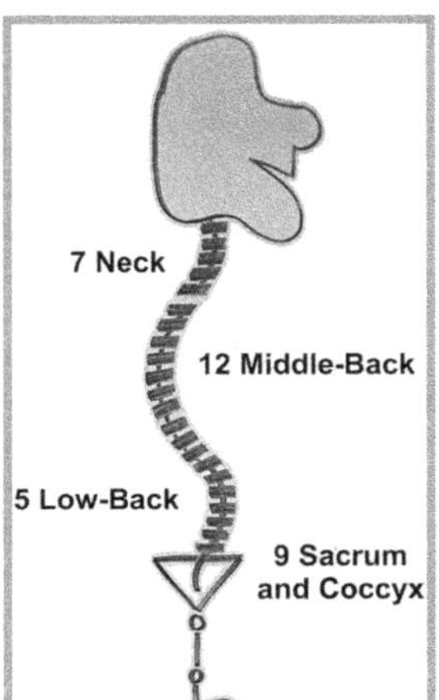

33 Bones—4 Parts

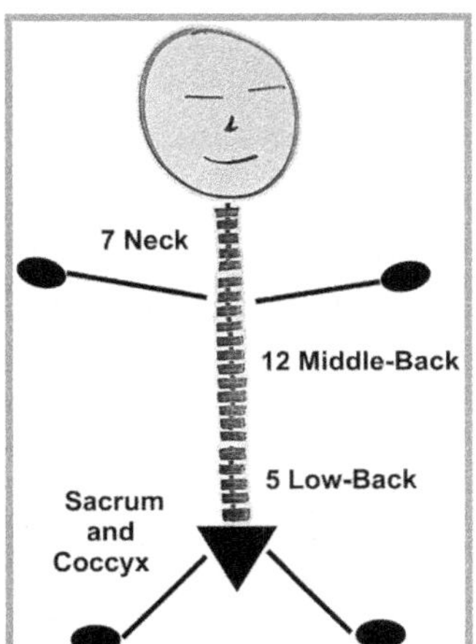

Vertically Straight Alignment

A Good Back Is Vertically Straight

The Good Back has a Vertically Straight Alignment. If you look at the front view of the skeletal figure, you can see that its 33 bones are stacked solidly and squarely, one on top of the other, in a straight line. This stacked and straight alignment gives the backbone **strength** to withstand the stress and pressure from body weight (load) and gravity's constant pull. However, if any bone isn't perfectly lined up with the one above and below it, physical stress will weaken that part. Scoliosis is an example.

SCOLIOSIS is a condition of the backbone that occurs when the Vertically Straight Alignment shifts into a single or double curvature. Fearing the weakened parts will eventually "buckle" under physical stress, bracing and surgery are the usual treatments. I would encourage those with this condition to follow *The Bad Back To Good Back Method* (Step 7, Restore The Balance).

A Good Back Has 4 Curves

The Good Back has 4 curves; 2 Master (neck and low-back) and 2 Servant (middle-back and sacrum). Appropriately named, the **stability** of the Master Curves DETERMINES the stability of the Servant Curves. In other words, the neck and low-back curves are MORE important.

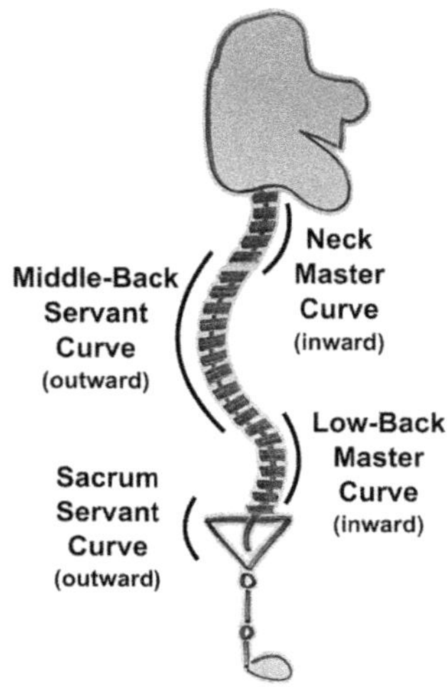

4—Curve Alignment

If you look at the side profile of the skeletal figure, you can see the Master Curves face *inward,* and the Servant Curves face *outward.* This alternating curvy pattern looks like a large *spring* and allows the backbone to act like one, too. Walking, running, jumping, dancing, skiing, and any other physical activity we can "dish out" will challenge the backbone's 4 curves to absorb physical stress and spring back (recoil).

Some of the best examples of a springy backbone can be found on America's Funniest Videos®. They are clips of people who have fallen off their bike, horse, or chair but, seemingly uninjured, get back up and walk away like nothing ever happened. WE laugh, but THEY should thank their backbone's 4 curves for acting like a spring, absorbing the impact, and rebounding!

Curve Physics

The alternating curves clearly give the backbone its **springy-ness**, but they also offer **strength** and **stability**. Physics tells us that the arc shape is one of the strongest and most stable structural shapes. The Delicate Arch at Arches National Park in Utah, the Gateway Arch in St. Louis, and the Arc de Triumph in Paris are well-known arches. These arc-shaped structures are strong and stable because their physical load has been equally distributed around their "arc-shaped curve" instead of concentrating at any one point. Similarly, the 4 *arc-shaped curves* of the back are strongest and most stable when the "load" each must carry is equally distributed around their curve. Here's how the concept plays out.

- **Neck Curve:** Equally distributes the *weight* of the head onto each of the 7 bones and 6 discs.
- **Middle-Back Curve:** Equally distributes the *weight* of the head, neck, and shoulders onto each of its 12 bones and 12 discs.
- **Low-Back Curve:** Equally distributes the *weight* of the head, neck, shoulders, and middle-back onto each of its 5 bones and 5 discs.
- **Sacrum Curve:** Equally distributes the *weight* of the upper body onto its 9 semi-fused and fused bones.

Lou's Back And Butt

Sadly, most people never consider whether the backbone has curves or not. Still, others believe the back is supposed to be absolutely straight. This is especially true if their mother scolded them to "straighten up" whenever they slouched or their yoga teacher encouraged them to flatten their back on their mat.

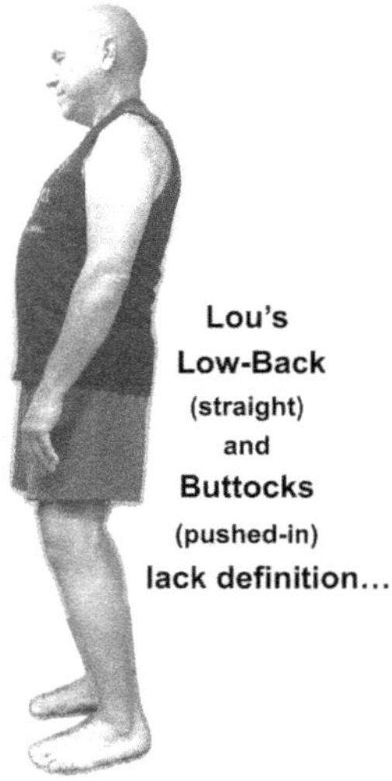
Lou's
Low-Back
(straight)
and
Buttocks
(pushed-in)
lack definition...

That was Lou. He was convinced his low-back was supposed to be straight, and he was proud he could get it to flatten completely on the floor during yoga. Lou was an active sixty-year-old who had both hips replaced and, to manage his low-back problems, attended three hot yoga classes weekly. He was anxious to tell me how yoga helped him avoid back surgery, but I was more concerned with Lou's straight lower back. Gazing at how his low-back bones and buttocks lacked definition, I surmised his Master Curve was pretty straight.

JoAnne's Experiment

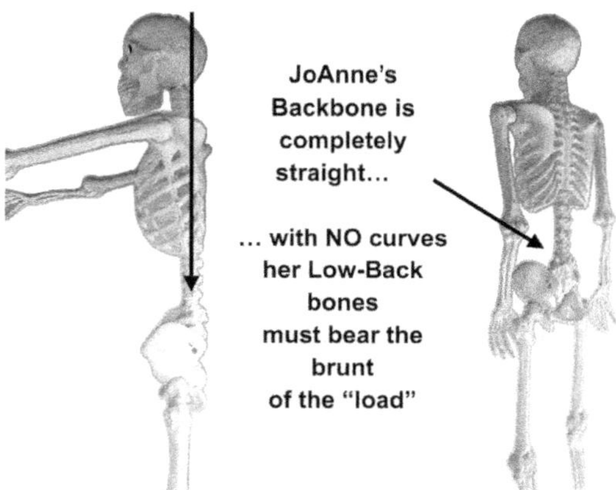

Let's continue talking about "curve physics." Take a look at JoAnne, the skeleton. *Can you see that her backbone is completely straight (no curves)?* Now, imagine I'm using both my hands to push straight down on top of her skull while applying a **good amount of force**. *What part of JoAnne's back would be affected by my push?*

The force from my downward push SHOULD BE equally distributed onto ALL 4 curves, but because JoAnne's back doesn't have them, her low-back bones receive **most** of the stress. In the short-term, this experiment wouldn't bother her low-back; however, if she had to endure me pushing on her head for years and years (like gravity), the bones are apt to buckle, and the discs could bulge. Statistics say most *bulging discs* occur within the low-back bones (L4-L5, L5-S1). Coincidently, that's where Lou's back problems were located.

GET TO KNOW THE OTHER PARTS

The backbone's curvy parts were designed to be strong, stable, and springy, but they are NOT the only parts. Take a peek at the skeleton's head and feet; they curve *outward* like the Servant Curves, and his knees curve *inward* like the Master Curves. This alternating *inward* and *outward* curvy pattern gives the skeletal structure "balance" and helps it function like a "whole body spring." *Now, tell me, is that not the* ***coolest thing*** *you've ever learned about your body?!*

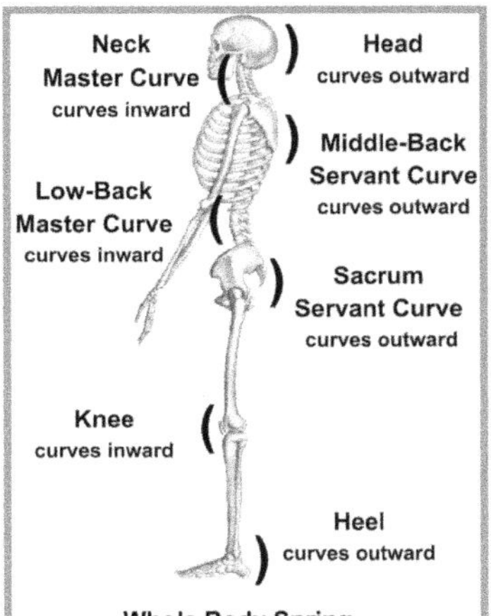

Whole Body Spring

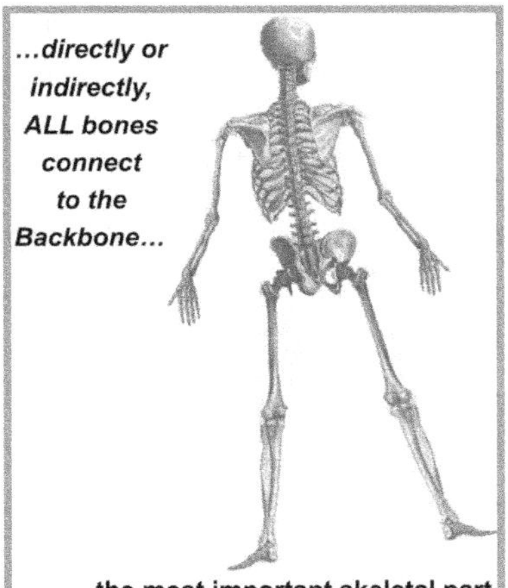

...the most important skeletal part

Here's something else we never think about… the backbone is like a tree trunk, and the "other bones" are like its branches. To the tips of the fingers and toes, every bone connects (directly or indirectly) to the backbone, making the backbone a very important skeletal part—probably the most.

In Other Words… Whatever direction the backbone (tree trunk) moves will affect (its branches) the skull, ribs, and pelvic bones because they are **directly attached** to the backbone.

That Is To Say… If they don't move too well, the sternum, jaw, arms, legs, and shoulder blades won't either because they **directly attach** to the skull, ribs, and pelvic bones.

Put Another Way… *Who can be blamed for hand problems?* Start at the wrist, go to the shoulder, clavicle, and sternum, which are held in place by several ribs that **directly attach** to the backbone. Voila, hand problems are the backbone's fault!

Who's At Fault… *If someone has TMJ?* Look to the jaw joints, which **directly attach** to the skull, that sit on top of Atlas (neck bone #1), and *TMJ…* is the backbone's fault!

Who's Responsible… *For bunions?* Start at the big toe, go to the ankle, knee, hip, and pelvic joints, that **directly attach** to the sacrum, and you guessed it… *bunions* are the backbone's fault!

When In Doubt… It's the backbone's fault.

The Good Back Dance Song

Do you remember the "Skeleton Dance Song?" You probably sang it as a child; its lyrics and tune are quite catchy…

> ♫ *The foot bone's connected to the leg bone… The leg bone's connected to the knee bone… The knee bone's connected to the thigh bone… Doin' the skeleton dance!* ♫

Here's my version, which highlights everything you've just learned about the Good Back. It's sung to the same melody:

♫ *The head, ribs, and pelvis... directly connect to the... backbone*
The jaw, arms, legs, and shoulder blades... indirectly connect to the... backbone
These ***skeletal parts****... require a* ***s-t-a-b-l-e****... backbone*
The Vertically Straight Alignment... give the backbone... ***s-t-r-e-n-g-t-h***
The 4 Curve Alignment.... give the backbone... ***s-t-a-b-i-l-i-t-y***
The alternating curves... give the backbone... ***s-p-r-i-n-g-y-n-e-s-s***
A strong, stable, and springy backbone... makes... the skeleton dance! ♫

Okay, it's cheeky, but in all seriousness, here's how the concept plays out...

The backbone, good or bad, can influence the "other bones" similarly, the "other bones" can influence the back. For this reason, you MUST learn what a Good Back looks like so you can easily recognize a Bad Back.

HOW TO RECOGNIZE A GOOD BACK

It's time to talk about how to recognize a Good Back. Now that you understand the backbone influences the "other bones," we can evaluate the "other bones" to recognize a Good Back. Before we can proceed, we **MUST** agree to:

Refer... To the neck, middle-back, low-back, and sacrum as *backbone parts*, and refer to the "other bones" as *skeletal parts.*

See... The skeletons are standing in *The Good Back Type*, just as nature designed you and me to stand: upright, tall, straight, and proud with our heads held high. **See images 1A, 1B.**

Recognize... The skeletal structure of EVERY human being should naturally stand in *The Good Back Type.* **See images 1C, 1D.**

Define... *The Good Back Type* to be the natural (not forced) standing alignment of a person's skeletal parts.

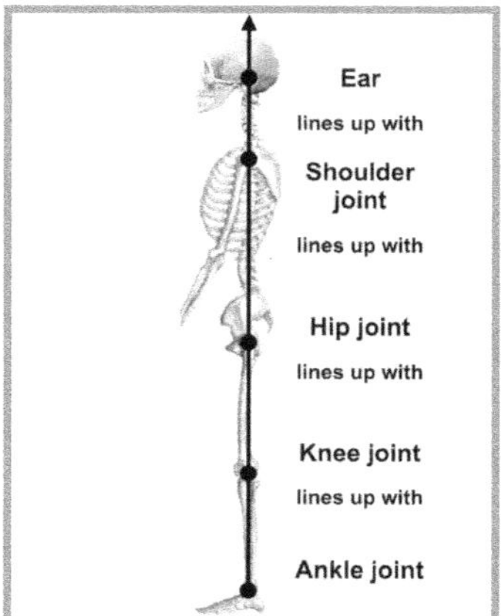

The Good Back Type
(Image 1A)

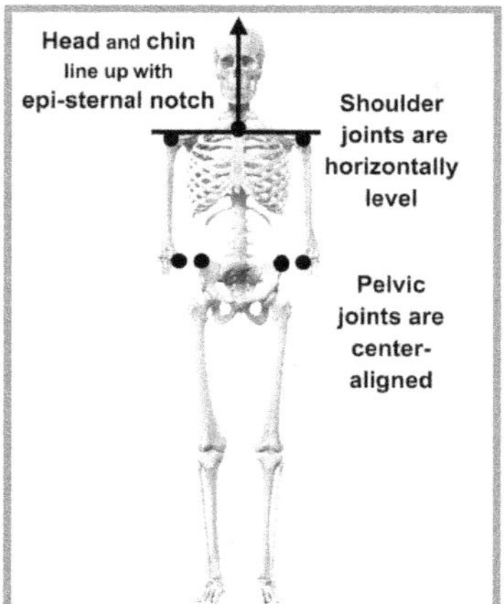

The Good Back Type
(Image 1B)

The Good Back Type can be confirmed when you look at a person's side profile and see that their ear, shoulder, hip, knee, and ankle joints line up. When those **skeletal parts** line up, it's a good indication that their **backbone parts** (neck, middle-back, low-back, sacrum) have a 4 Curve Alignment.

When you look directly at a person (front view), their head (and chin) lines up with their episternal notch (bony groove under the throat), their shoulders are horizontally level, and their pelvis is center-aligned. When those **skeletal parts** line up, it's a good indication that their **backbone parts** (neck, middle-back, low-back, sacrum) have a Vertically Straight Alignment.

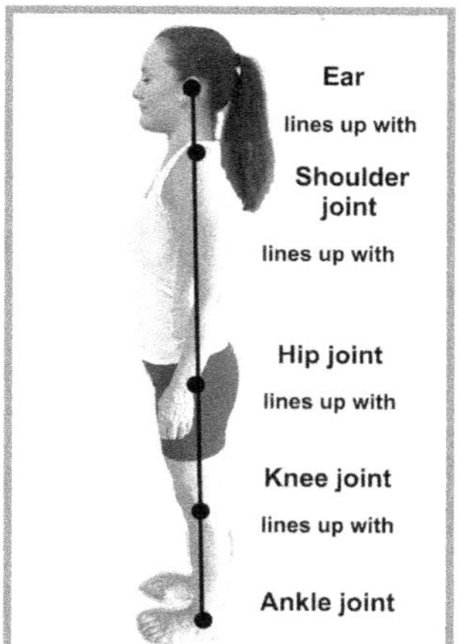

The Good Back Type
(Image 1C)

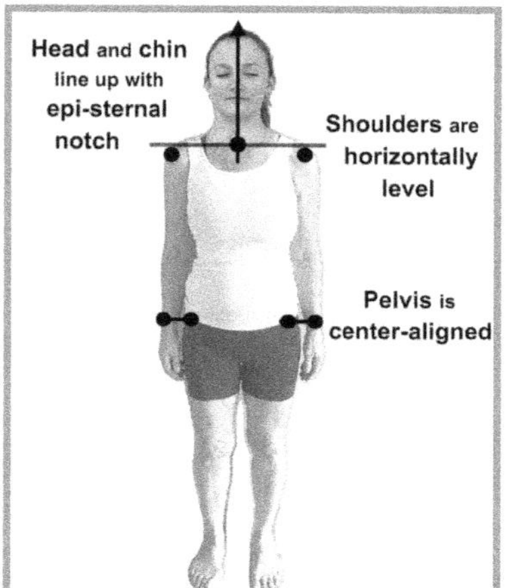

The Good Back Type
(Image 1D)

Q: *What causes a Good Back to become a Bad Back?*

A: When the straight and/or curvy alignment of a backbone part has been compromised.

Q: *How will you know you have a Bad Back?*

A: Your skeletal parts DO NOT line up when you stand (unless you force them).

The Good Back In A Nutshell

We've officially concluded what it means to have a Good Back. A Vertically Straight and 4 Curve Alignment are the foundational components necessary for the back to function as a strong, stable, and springy structure.

When the backbone isn't straight and doesn't have curves, that's a Bad Back. It's the problem—the whole problem—and nothing but back problems. It's what went wrong with your back when you first started having problems, and it will cause you additional back problems if you don't **restore** the straight and **restore** the curves.

It's not your fault... the blame must be placed on educational institutions, mainstream medical, and alternative therapy practitioners who continually overlook the backbone's Vertically Straight and 4 Curve Alignment as the REAL reason for back problems. They look everywhere else and blame everything BUT a bent alignment or curveless curves. Yet, the backbone's straight and curvy alignment isn't radical; it's not complicated—it's just physics. If **everyone** would just focus on straightening the parts of the back that need to be straightened or curving the parts that need to be curved, you wouldn't need to read this book.

That is WHY I've written this self-guided manual for YOU. You are about to learn how to take your Bad Back, make it straight, and give it curves until it becomes a Good Back. This book promises to guide you to **restore** your backbone's Vertically Straight and 4 Curve Alignment because that's the only way you are going to get permanent relief from your back problems.

STEP 2: FIND OUT WHAT MAKES A GOOD BACK GO BAD

Force is a physical law we are all familiar with, but we don't think much about it. Yet, it can cause a straight backbone to become bent or curves to straighten. In this step, you will learn how **quick** and **slow forces** are responsible for taking a Good Back and making it Bad.

QUICK FORCES MAKE BAD BACKS

Have you ever slipped on ice, tumbled down the stairs, crashed your car, tripped on a loose carpet, or been involved in a sport-related collision? If yes, then some part of your skeletal structure was probably affected by that sudden impact, and you experienced a *quick force*. When I was in clinical practice, I routinely asked new patients if they remembered having an accident, even dating as far back as their childhood. Most could recall at least one.

> *... I can't believe I totally forgot I was thrown from a motorcycle when I was in my twenties... My husband reminded me of the time I was holding a basket of laundry, stepped on a toy, and slid down the basement stairs... I remember a football game in which I was tackled so hard that the wind got knocked out of me... The fall on my back while I brushed snow off the car totally escaped my memory... Looking back twenty-five years ago, I rolled my jeep but walked away from that accident without a scratch...*

When a *quick force* meets an arm, leg, head, or butt, it can happen in the blink of an eye and often leaves visible signs like a bruise or fracture. That's when it's easy to assume it was the only body part affected. However, consider another part of the skeletal structure most likely stressed by a quick force. Hint... *the foot bone connects to the leg bone...* all the way back to the backbone.

In other words, a *quick force* impact may "act" on one part of the skeletal structure, but because every part is connected to the backbone, it's likely to cause stress and movement to any of the backbone's movable, semi-fused, or fused bones.

The Straw That Broke The Camel's Back

Charles was an elderly man whose upper body was, quite literally, folded in half. He believed the accident that caused him to be "slumped over" occurred when he ran to catch a bus, tripped on the curb, and fell to the ground on his side. Charles sustained several broken ribs and couldn't stand up straight from that day forward. He angrily stated, *I can't get around without my walker, and I'm in constant pain unless I'm sitting in my recliner. I wouldn't be in this condition if I hadn't tripped trying to get on that bus!*

Charles was hell-bent on blaming the accident, but I wasn't convinced a single stumble and fall would cause him to become crippled. Searching for additional clues, I questioned Charles and found what I was looking for when he recalled multiple accidents in his youth.

Charles' first accident occurred at age eight when he fell out of an apple tree. When he was twelve, he fell out of the hay loft. Charles' third incident happened when he was twenty-two and jumped out of an empty box car while the train was moving. Years after his train jump, Charles developed a limp, but it wasn't until he was in his fifties that he noticed how crookedly he stood. Then, in a mournful tone, expressed this realization: *It just never occurred to me that I was in such rough shape decades before I tripped; now I understand it was the straw that broke my back!*

Many of you can relate to Charles' story and recall at least one or more accidents. Maybe you've never considered them a contributing factor because they happened long before your back problems became noticeable. After giving some thought to your history, here's hoping you can easily say, *Yep, that's the one!*

When a *quick force* acts on the back, bones can be abruptly moved from their Vertically Straight or 4 Curve Alignment to an incorrect alignment. This is referred to as a misalignment, and bones that misalign can do so individually or as a whole. There are two types of misalignments: *Shift-and-Separate* and *All-Shift-Together*.

SHIFT-AND-SEPARATE MISALIGNMENT

This type of misalignment occurs when a **bone** shifts and **separates** from the bone **above** and/or **below** it. The direction of the separation can be forward, backward, or sideways and may include several bones, not just one. The back is likely to have this type of misalignment if it encountered an intense compressive stress (like from lifting weights), a violent impact (like from whiplash), or a direct blow (like from a fall or hit). These examples could produce enough force to cause one or more bones to Shift-and-Separate, which would affect their stacked alignment (bones no longer stack one on top of the other solidly and squarely). A Shift-and-Separate Misalignment can ONLY be identified with an X-ray or MRI.

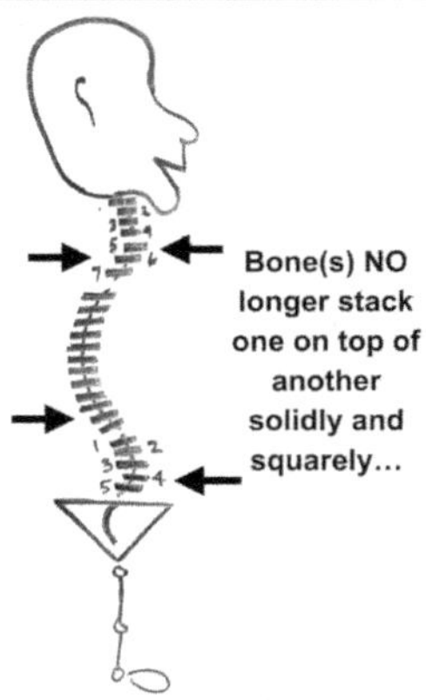

Shift-and-Separate Misalignment

(Image 2A)

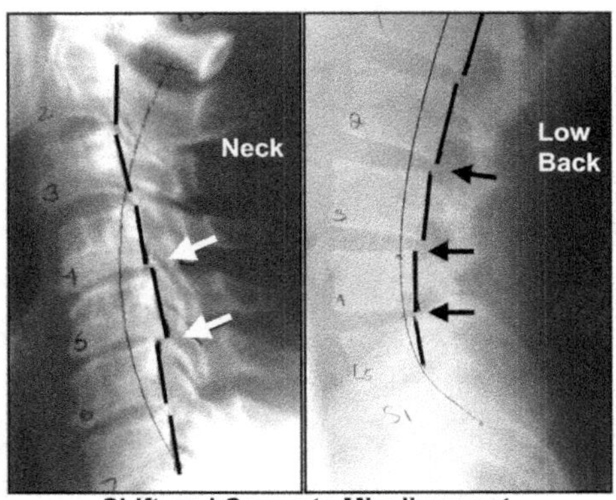

Shift-and-Separate Misalignment

(Image 2B)

ALL-SHIFT-TOGETHER MISALIGNMENT

An All-Shift-Together Misalignment occurs when one or more **parts** of the backbone **shift** from their curved or straight alignment to an incorrect alignment. The bones can shift forward, backward, or sideways but **always together** and in the **same direction.** Slow forces (gravity) or a high-impact accident (whiplash) could produce enough force to cause an entire backbone part (neck, middle-back, low-back, sacrum) to All-Shift-Together. A **Structural Evaluation** as taught by *The Bad Back To Good Back Method* (Step 6) and weight-bearing X-ray films can easily detect this type of misalignment, but NOT an MRI, motion palpation, or neuro-thermal scans.

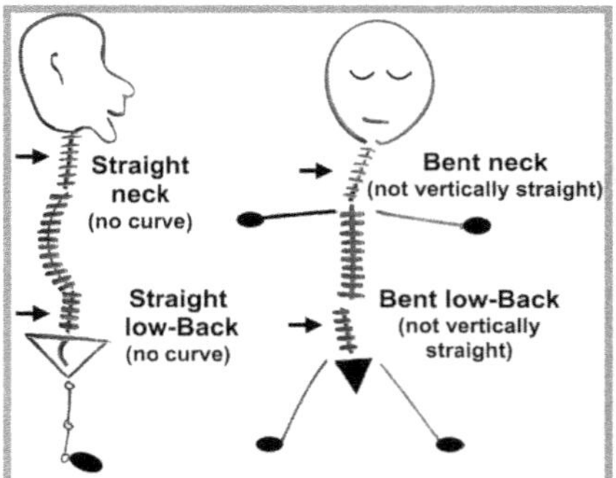

All-Shift-Together Misalignment

(Image 2C)

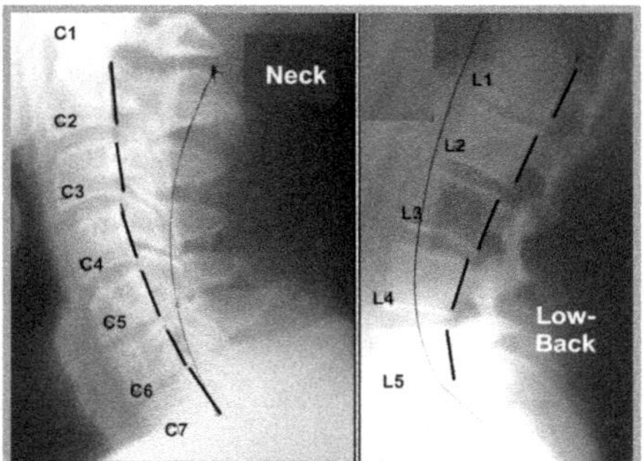

All-Shift-Together Misalignment

(Image 2D)

Johnny's Obituary

Several years ago, before I opened a new office, I thought it would be easier to educate patients if I used a full-sized skeleton to demonstrate the backbone. We've all seen a paper skeleton around Halloween, but to see a skeleton up close and study how all the bones connect to the backbone was a 3-D experience I thought patients would appreciate. I searched high and low until I found a man-sized skeleton from a manufacturer in another country.

When the box arrived, it was too big to bring inside the house, so I let my very enthusiastic fourteen-year-old son, Justin, put it together on the back deck. About thirty minutes later, the skeleton was assembled, wholly held up by a steel rod that went from its skull through its butt and inserted into a base on wheels. This skeleton was perfect in every way, EXCEPT, it wasn't standing up straight. It sort of leaned forward and a bit to the Left, so its shoulder hung low and looked like a rag doll.

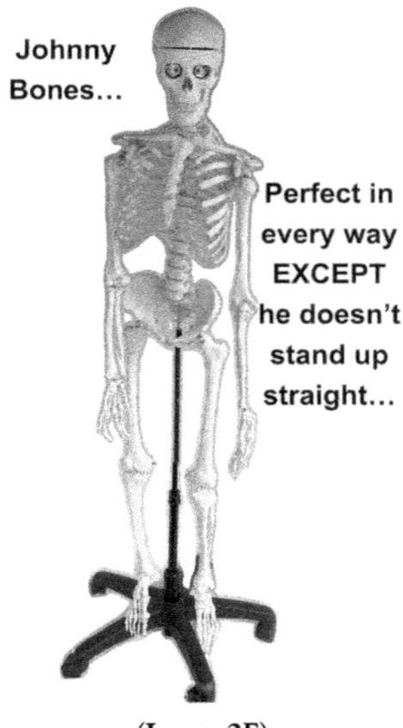

(Image 2E)

Guessing Justin didn't follow the directions and probably missed a screw or two, we frantically searched the box for the instructions. Among the styrofoam and wrappings, we stumbled upon a postcard. At first, I thought it was a QC (quality control) label signifying all parts and pieces were in the box, but as I reviewed it more closely, I realized it was this skeleton's obituary. It read:

This is Mr. John Ossein. He was a sixty-seven-year-old male of Polish descent who never recovered from whiplash complications after a cement truck smashed into his car. Johnny was riddled with arthritis from multiple herniated discs in his neck that caused him twenty-five years of pain, suffering, and several unsuccessful neck surgeries (his last was fatal). Johnny was a good man and dearly loved, and because his last name means bone, he was known as Johnny Bones. Johnny's last wish to his family was to donate his body to science, and requested glass eyes be made to replicate his own baby blues, a forewarning to his researchers that he'd be watching over them.

Stunned to learn this, Justin and I **stared** at the skeleton. That's when it hit us. Johnny wasn't a plastic skeleton after all; his structure was the remains of a real human being! Then, it all made sense. Johnny wasn't leaning because of a missing bolt or screw but from his motor vehicle accident. I imagined the *quick force* impact caused Johnny's body to be thrown forward, and that's how his skeletal structure remained for ***the... rest... of... his... life.***

Johnny's Whiplash

If I had to guess, I'd say Johnny must have hit his head on the steering wheel pretty hard to produce multiple *herniated discs.* No doubt, when his car was hit, the quick force impact threw his head forward, and his neck bones followed. Take a peek at Johnny's neck curve; it doesn't exist at all; in fact, it's completely straight. Car accidents (even minor ones) can force one or more parts of the back to All-Shift-Together to become misaligned and remain stuck in the direction they were thrown. But an impact doesn't always need to be fast and furious to cause bones to shift—it can happen slowly.

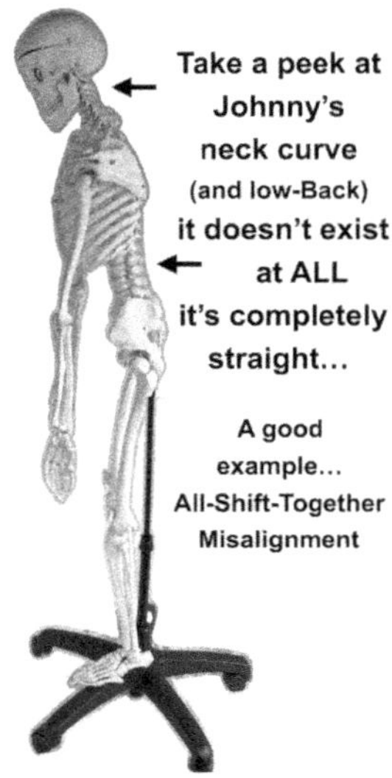

(Image 2F)

SLOW FORCES MAKE BAD BACKS

Do you sit hunched over your computer at the office, at the dining room table, and more than you'd like to admit, on the couch? When you look down at your phone (average 300+ min/day), does your head and neck tilt forward? Are you a driver for a shipping, bus, or postal service and spend countless hours on your rump?

If you aren't sitting, maybe you stand hunched over a task or activity for hours at a time. Whatever your daily activities, I'm willing to bet you subject some part of your skeletal structure to a fixed position for an extended period, which means you've experienced a **slow force**. Holding any body part in a sustained position or imposing a repetitive activity are everyday stresses that slowly force bones to shift and ever so gradually, a backbone part gets pulled until those bones All-Shift-Together. That's when a curve straightens or a straight part becomes bent.

I can't tell you how many patients have questioned whether the decades they spent sitting at a desk, kneeling to lay brick sidewalks, or standing over a cash register caused their back problems. If they denied having any *quick force* accidents, I would explain that the repetitive activities and sustained positions their skeletal structure endured every day while they worked, played, sat, or slept had more of an impact on their backbones than any one traumatic event.

When a slow force acts on a Good Back, bones can gradually move from their Vertically Straight or 4 Curve Alignment to an incorrect alignment. Remember, the two types of misalignments are Shift-and-Separate and All-Shift-Together, and they are responsible for taking a Good Back and making it bad.

BULGING DISC is a condition of the backbone that's often the result of a slow compressive force placed on bones and discs over a long period of time. The cushion-like disc material reacts to the stress by either disintegrating or slowly bulging out between the bones like a squashed jelly donut. This is why a person may never feel their *bulging disc;* it squeezed out **ever… so… slowly.** Some bulges don't appear until years after an accident. It's been said that more than half of the population walks around with at least one asymptomatic *bulging disc* (Step 5, *Bulging* and *Herniated Discs).*

Joe and The Johnny Jump

Joe was a forty-three-year-old software engineer who came to my office because he thought he was becoming paralyzed. I located an L4-L5 *spondylolisthesis* on his low-back X-rays that he didn't know he had (which is typical of this condition). When I questioned him, Joe couldn't recall a past accident or injury that could account for his condition and confirmed he had never played sports.

Me: *That's good to know. I can rule out quick forces as the possible cause of your Shift-and-Separate Misalignment because you didn't partake in contact sports during your youth, which is often the cause. Do you know anything about being placed in a Johnny Jump when you were a baby?*

Joe: *A what?*

Me: *It's a hanging bouncy swing for babies that hooks onto a door-jam molding. Do you know if your parents put you in one of those as a baby?*

Joe: *I'll ask my Mom tonight.*

Joe's low-back condition, where L4 had shifted and separated forward of L5, would occasionally cause his legs to go numb. Over the years, he noticed they lacked strength and felt heavy when he walked the three flights of stairs to his apartment. A couple of days after our consultation, Joe excitedly walked into our office because he had the answer to my question.

Joe: *My mother not only confirmed putting me in a Johnny Jump but a baby walker, too. She laughed, remembering that I was full of energy and those toys were the only things that entertained me.*

Me: *This helps explain your case. When you sat in the Johnny Jump and bounced, bounced, bounced, then stood to walk, walk, walk in the baby walker, the part of your backbone that was stressed was the L4-L5 joint.*

Despite being baby-soft cartilage, the impact was enough to weaken the area. Over the next forty years, L4 slowly shifted forward to affect the nerve roots and cause neurological problems.

Joe: *Do I have to worry about becoming paralyzed?*

Me: *You will learn how to restore your low-back Master Curve in Step 7, and as a result, your nerves should gradually resume normal function, but left alone, surgery may be your only recourse.*

SPONDYLOLISTHESIS (SPAHN-di-low-less-THEE-sis) is a Shift-and-Separate Misalignment condition that can affect any movable backbone but most commonly affects low-back bones L4-L5 or L5-S1. In Joe's case, his *spondylolisthesis* started with the repetitive action of bouncing in his Johnny Jump as a baby. As he aged, his bones continued to move in that same direction (**slow force**) until low-back bone #4 slipped so far forward on bone #5 that it began to affect his L4-L5 spinal nerve root, which was evidenced by the paralysis he was experiencing in his legs. Check out Joe's post-X-ray, which demonstrates that restoration is possible.

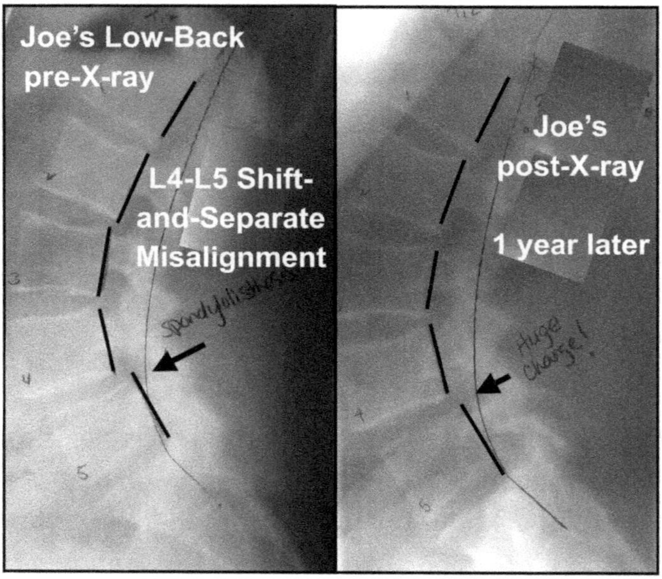

Recalling your accident history can put your mind at ease just to know that your back problem started with a *quick force* impact. Still, back problems that CAN'T be linked to any accident or injury are likely due to slow and gradual forces, quietly nudging the bones from stability. The Good Back goes bad when bones Shift-and-Separate or All-Shift-Together to compromise the Vertically Straight and 4 Curve Alignment. In some cases, the misalignments can affect the soft wiring.

WHEN THE BACK GOES BAD IT CAN AFFECT THE SOFT WIRING

With a basic understanding of the Nervous System and how it's "wired," you'll be better able to recognize how a Bad Back can cause all sorts of nerve problems. The brain and spinal cord are two of the most important organs of your entire body. They are completely **encased** and **protected** by the skull and backbone. The brain s-q-u-e-e-z-e-s itself through a hole (Foramen Magnum) at the bottom of the skull, thus becoming the brainstem, then continues through Atlas (neck bone #1) and Axis (neck bone #2) to run the length of your backbone as the spinal cord.

Imagine —> The waitress has just placed a chocolate milkshake on the table before you. *Yum!* You pull the shake closer, put the straw in your mouth and begin to suck the shake up through the straw (*OMG, that milkshake is SO good).* That's precisely how the spinal cord (milkshake) fits within the backbone (straw); it's a really tight fit.

Branching off the spinal cord are spinal nerve roots that branch again and again, all the way to the tips of your fingers and toes. This soft wiring is your neurological system, and it's the route your brain takes to "talk" to your body. Communication begins when the brain tells the body's systems how to function. Nerve impulses travel lightning fast from the brain, down the spinal cord, out the nerve roots to all parts of the body (to send information), and then back to the brain again (to receive information). This incoming and outgoing communication is why you don't have to think about processing your food, pumping your blood, ensuring your lungs carry oxygen, removing your hand from a hot burner, or engaging your muscles to walk.

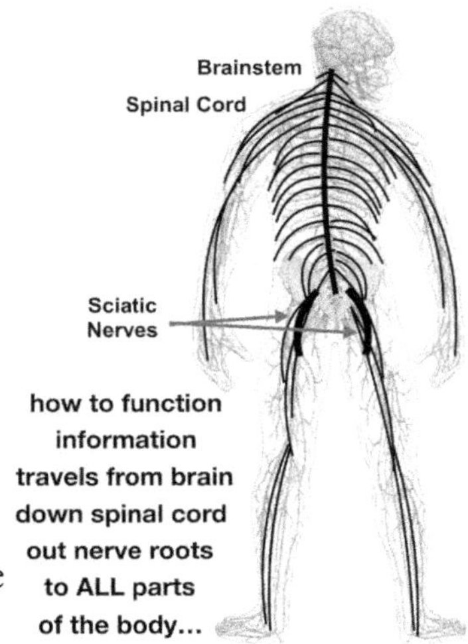

(Image 2G)

Q: *Could this "how to function" communication be affected if the backbone's straight or curvy alignment were compromised (misaligned)?*

A: Yes. There's no wiggle room between the bones (straw) and spinal cord or nerve roots (milkshake). When bones shift, they create pressure (like a bend in your straw), which alters incoming and outgoing information.

Peter's Cold Hands

Peter came to our office with neck pain and cold hands. He complained that his hands would go numb and become terribly cold while driving his car or lawn tractor, and especially when playing golf. Peter's neck

X-rays revealed a reversed curve, the faulty part of his backbone. After implementing the BB2GB Method for three months, Peter reported, "*I can't recall when it happened, but my hands aren't icicles anymore, and I'm so excited that I don't need to wear gloves while I mow the lawn or play golf.*"

To my surprise, Peter had *Raynaud's Syndrome* and never mentioned it (he didn't realize his condition had a clinical name). For years, he and his wife had been planning to move south due to this problem but didn't want to go because their children and grandchildren lived nearby. Peter was my first successful encounter with a nerve-related condition, but one that proves how the sensory part of the nerves can malfunction when the neck curve is reversed.

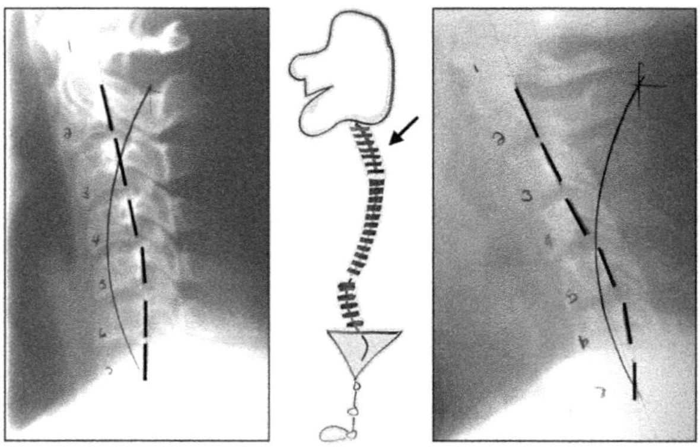

Reversed Neck Master Curve
(Image 2H)

RAYNAUD'S SYNDROME is a condition similar to *carpal tunnel* that affects the sensory part of the nerves supplying the hands and fingers, so temperature changes are the usual complaint. Onset is believed to be genetics and emotional stress, but every case of *Raynaud's* that "presented" to our office had a reversed neck curve, which suggests that *Raynaud's* is more likely the result of physical stress.

CARPAL TUNNEL SYNDROME is a nerve-related condition that affects the motor part of the nerves supplying the hands and fingers. Decreased function is the usual complaint, and it's often blamed on *nerve compression* caused by prolonged or repetitive hand/wrist activities. Let's trace the nerves from under the sheath at the wrist (where surgery occurs), up the arm to the connecting nerve bundle, then onto their spinal roots (sandwiched between neck bones C5-6, C6-C7, C7-T1). *Could this syndrome result from neck bones that have shifted forward and compressed the spinal nerve roots?* Yes, and that makes *carpal tunnel* the backbone's fault.

PINCHED NERVE is a condition that occurs when spinal nerve roots experience pressure from the backbone and become irritated and inflamed. Nerve roots DON'T like to be pinched or pulled, and if they are, they will respond with a variety of sensations; burning, stabbing, throbbing, and radiating pain, numbness, tingling, pins and needles, and temperature changes. Those nerves may lose their ability to function correctly, and that's how neurological conditions arise. *Pinched nerves* are *compressed nerves*, so both are the backbone's fault.

A Riddle For What's Ahead

When the Good Back goes BAD, faulty ***backbone parts*** *MUST be blamed…*

And not many know that's the GAME…

To "find" the compromised parts, our ***skeletal parts*** *give us CLUES…*

Most "clues" are obvious, while some are not, but every "clue" suggests the damaged PART…

Detective skills are few–steady eyes and a guess or two–are sure to guide the quest, and restoration is up to YOU…

Part II

BAD BACK SYNDROME REVEALED

STEP 3: LEARN AND OBSERVE THE OBVIOUS BAD BACK SIGNS

In this step, you will learn about the Obvious Bad Back Signs that create Bad Back Syndrome Types (Step 5) and affect the backbone's 4 curves. The Not-So-Obvious Bad Back Signs create *Quirky's* (Step 4) and affect the backbone's straight alignment. *Bowling Ball Head, Cold Shoulders, HunchBack Shoulders, Pelvic Thrust 'n' Tilt,* and *Pelvic Back-Ender w/ Dip* are the Obvious Bad Back Signs named after the faulty **skeletal part** they represent. Because the "obvious signs" affect the backbone's curvy alignment, they can be quickly and easily recognized when you look at a person's side profile. Plan on having fun spotting "obvious signs" because everyone has at least three of them!

> ***BAD BACK SYNDROME*** is a condition of the backbone characterized by several faulty parts of the skeletal structure (head, shoulders, pelvis) that produce Obvious Bad Back Signs and Not-So-Obvious Bad Back Signs (*Quirky's*). These "signs" identify the faulty parts of the backbone (neck, middle-back, low-back, sacrum) that have compromised strength, stability, and springy-ness. *Bad Back Syndrome Types* are derived from combinations of Obvious Bad Back Signs.

The Demonstration

Several years ago, my family and I gathered at our annual Christmas Eve party at my brother-in-law's bowling alley. Since bowling was the theme, we split into teams and chose a ball, (I picked two). As the games ensued, I used the heavier green ball (14 lbs.) for my first throw, which occasionally produced a strike. I followed up with the lighter pink one

(10 lbs.), which occasionally produced a spare. For game three, my arm was getting tired, so I used the pink ball exclusively, and my team finished third, which I thought was pretty good, considering we only bowl once a year. As I returned the balls to the shelf, I suddenly realized my attachment to the pink one and dashed off to find my brother-in-law. With a dramatic whine, I held the ball tight and pleaded with him to let me take it home.

He responded, *"If you want one so badly, why don't you buy one?"*

I smiled, shook my head and replied, *"I don't want a bowling ball to BOWL with… I want one to use for my demonstrations! If I can have this old ball, my presentations will be much better, and it won't cost me a cent because you'll* ***gift*** *it to me."*

Now, my pretty pink ball has a new purpose. At our Lunch 'n' Learns, my assistant Sarah would place the bowling bag at my feet while the curious crowd watched me unzip and reach in. Fingers in each hole, I'd lift the ball above my head and twirl it around like we were at a beauty contest. I'd ask, *Can anyone guess how much this ball weighs?* Eventually, I'd tell them it was 10 pounds if nobody guessed. Then, I'd ask for a volunteer to help me with a little weight competition.

When the volunteer arrived at my side, I'd hand them the ball and instruct them to hold it with their arms extended straight out. Then I'd make the offer: *If you can hold the bowling ball for 5 minutes without bending or lowering your arms, I'll give you this crisp $10 bill.* This is how it often played out: the weight of the ball would cause the volunteer's elbows to bend, and slowly the ball lowered toward the floor. Few people took my money because they couldn't hold their arms outstretched for the entire exercise. After they gave up, I'd ask them to bring the ball into their stomach, clench it tightly, and hold it there for as long as possible. *This is easy,* they'd say. *I could hold the ball like this all day long!*

The Point of the Demonstration

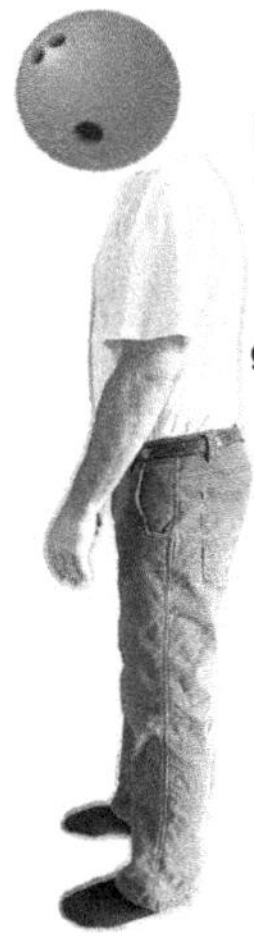
He complains the weight of his *Bowling Ball Head* gets heavy on his neck and shoulders...

Your head, like my bowling ball, weighs about 10 pounds. When it's sitting directly on top of your shoulders, in its natural alignment, your neck and shoulders can easily hold your head upright all day long without getting tired (like the volunteer holding the ball with the support of their stomach).

When your 10-pound head is extended forward (like the volunteer's outstretched arms), the weight of your head gets heavy on your neck and shoulders. That physical stress and strain can cause muscles to spasm, and a *tension headache* may develop.

> ***TENSION HEADACHE*** is a condition caused by physically stretched and strained neck and shoulder muscles. Muscles don't like to be stressed, and if the stress doesn't let up, they will spasm, fatigue, and become tense; hence, muscle tension. If you suffer from *migraines*, you probably already know that a *tension headache* "showed up" first.

(#1) *BOWLING BALL HEAD SIGN*

When a person's head shifts forward from its natural alignment, that is *Bowling Ball Head*. The head is the faulty part of the skeletal structure that influences the neck bones to shift forward to become the faulty part of the backbone. This Bad Back Sign is characterized by an outstretched head.

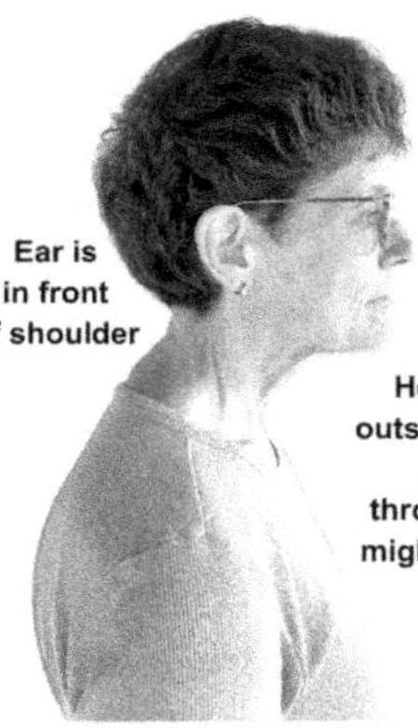

Bowling Ball Head Sign

Quick Glance —> The easiest way to discover if a person has *Bowling Ball Head Sign* is to observe that their ear doesn't line up with their shoulder; it's forward. Sometimes, the ear is just slightly in front of the shoulder, but if it's significant, you'll probably see their throat skin sag!

Bowling Ball Head Physics

The skull, Atlas (neck bone #1), and Axis (neck bone #2) are solely responsible for *Bowling Ball Head*. Follow the exercises below to understand how this plays out.

Try This —> Nod your head up and down several times, like the gesture "yes." This movement is possible because your skull joints ROCK on the Atlas joints.

Try This —> Slide your finger from the base of your skull down the neck until you feel a bone sticking out; that's the **tail of Axis**. Slide your finger upward into the "space" between the skull and Axis and press in; the **tail of Atlas** is way in there. Nod "yes" again (but exaggerate the movement) until you can feel the tail of Atlas ROLL into your finger.

Try This —> Rotate your head side to side several times, like the gesture "no." This movement is made possible because Atlas and Axis are bound together by a bony rod, so they move in unison.

Try This —> Drop your head (chin to chest). That movement just caused your skull to ROCK on Atlas, Atlas ROLLED with it, and Axis had to FOLLOW along.

Physics Explained

Approximately 150 times per day, you hold your head in a downward position. This repetitive action forces your skull, Atlas, and Axis to start the march forward, but don't forget, neck bones 3, 4, 5, and 6 will trail along because they All-Shift-Together. **See page 16, images 2C, 2D**. That is how *Bowling Ball Head* develops, and the neck curve straightens.

The problem with one compromised curve is that it will impact another. When the head and neck bones shift forward, they pull the middle-back bones and shoulders. This process is a simple game of "follow the leader," and it leads to another prominent Bad Back Sign: *Cold Shoulders.*

(#2) *COLD SHOULDERS SIGN*

When a person's shoulder girdle shifts forward from its natural alignment, that is *Cold Shoulders*. The shoulders are the faulty part of the skeletal structure that influences middle-back bones to shift forward to become the faulty part of the backbone. This Bad Back Sign is characterized by shoulders that have folded down and inward (like someone cold and shivering).

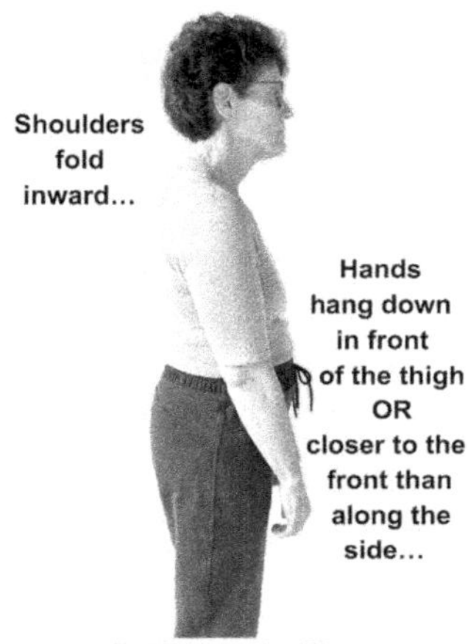

Cold Shoulder Sign

Quick Glance —> The easiest way to discover if a person has *Cold Shoulders Sign* is to observe whether their hands "hang down" in front of their thighs or closer to the front than along the side.

Shyness Looks Like *Cold Shoulders*

A father once approached me about his six-year-old daughter, Amy, who acted shy around everyone. *"It's concerning,"* Jeff said. *"She crouches her head, hunches her shoulders, and stares at the ground."* I responded, *"Amy's shyness may have long-term physical implications, especially because her skeletal structure is still developing. If she continues to hold her head, neck bones, middle-back bones, and shoulders in that "shy position" she's likely to have problems later in life. Essentially, she's changing the physical development of her shoulder joints by training them to fold down and in. I would advise you to go to Step 7 to learn how you can help her reverse that Cold Shoulders tendency, and I'm willing to bet she'll have fun molding right beside you."*

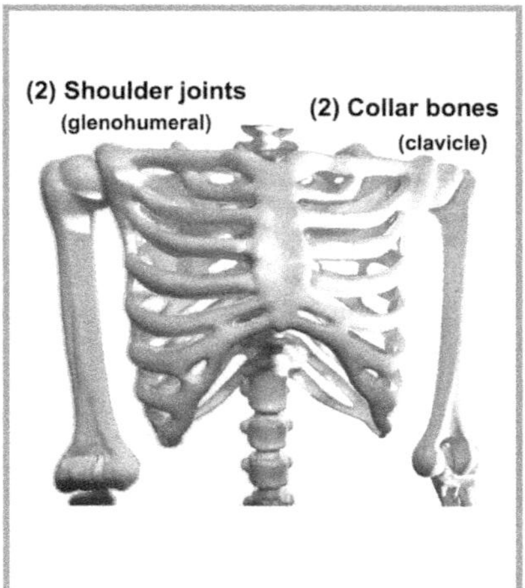

Shoulder Girdle (front view)
(Image 3A)

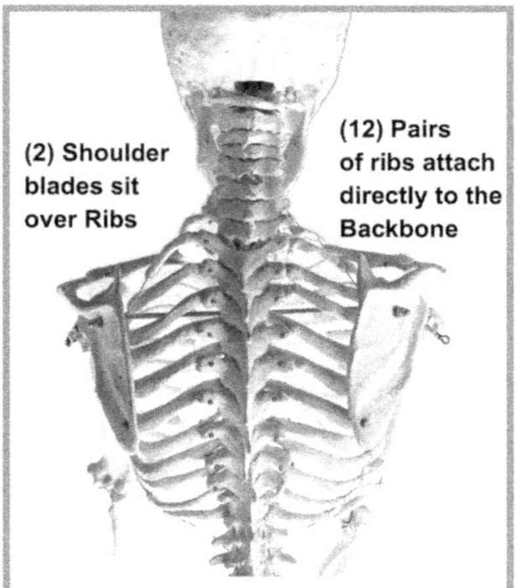

Shoulder Girdle (back view)
(Image 3B)

Shoulder Problems Explained

During clinical practice, when consulting with new patients, I always asked them if they had any *rotator cuff, frozen shoulder,* or other shoulder issues. These problems are relatively common, and few blame them on their faulty middle-back bones. With a quick anatomy lesson, shoulder problems become entirely clear.

To begin with: it may be helpful to know that the shoulders are NOT part of the backbone; their function is to operate WITH the backbone. Your shoulders, **aka** the shoulder girdle, consist of (2) collar bones (clavicle), (2) shoulder blades (scapula), and (2) shoulder joints (humerus). NONE of these "girdle joints" connect directly to the middle-back bones, but they interact closely with 12 ribs that do. When middle-back bones shift forward, backward, or off to the side, the ribs and "girdle joints" MUST follow. This "follow the leader" game alters the shoulder's natural alignment so that joint problems can arise.

Shoulder problems are pretty common among golfers, hockey players, bowlers, and tennis players (to name a few), who often have one shoulder that's more problematic. *Could that result from purposely dipping their dominant arm or shoulder more than the other to swing their club, stick, ball, or racket?* Yes, that repetitive activity makes the joint more susceptible to injury. In every case that "presented" to our office, the person's shoulder failed to function normally because they had *Cold Shoulders.*

If you have *shoulder problems,* take a look at your hand placement. Your hands should hang to the sides of your thighs when you stand. If they "hang down" in front of your thighs, your shoulders have rounded inward.

(#3) *HUNCHBACK SHOULDERS SIGN*

When a person's shoulder girdle shifts backward from its natural alignment, that is *HunchBack Shoulders.* The shoulders are the faulty part of the skeletal structure that influences middle-back bones to shift backward to become the faulty part of the backbone. In most cases, the shoulder joints will fold inward, which means the person with this sign ALSO has *Cold Shoulders.* This Bad Back Sign is characterized by an exaggerated middle-back that appears "hunched."

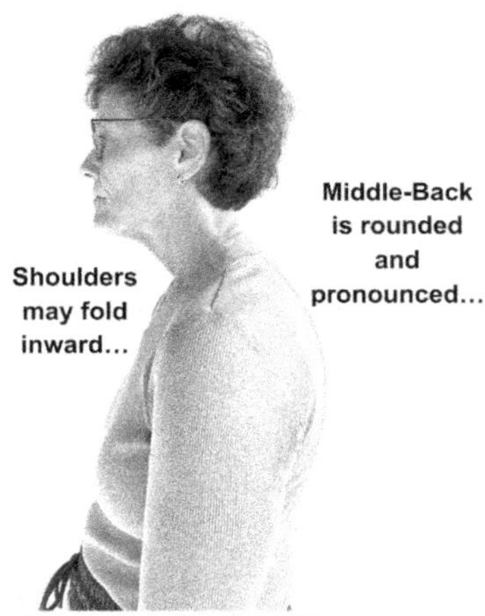

HunchBack Shoulder Sign

Quick Glance —> The easiest way to discover if a person has *HunchBack Shoulders Sign* is to observe a rounded and prominent middle-back (shoulder blade area). This pronounced appearance is especially noticeable as someone "sits back" on their middle-back.

Gabby's Shoulder Click

Gabby: *So I'm in yoga class, and you know how you bring your hands together at the top of your head? That's when I heard this "click" in my Right shoulder. It's been bothering me, I don't know, maybe a month or so, and I'm having a hard time raising and turning my arm during class. At first, I thought maybe I had* *injured my shoulder, you know, like lifting something heavy, but I haven't done anything unusual all summer. It's crunch time at work, and sometimes, I'm huddled over my computer for eight hours straight! When I get home, my neck and shoulders are achy, and several times a week, I wake up with a headache. But this "clicking noise" in my shoulder has me worried, especially because it's been a couple of months, and it's not going away. What do you think it is?*

I knew Gabby needed to understand the "clicking" in her shoulder joint was a mechanical problem, which meant I needed Johnny Bones. First, I showed her Johnny's straight neck **(See page 18, image 2F)** and explained that *Bowling Ball Head* can cause the neck and shoulders to be achy and stiff. She nodded with interest. Next, I pointed out how Johnny leaned forward, which pulled his shoulders down and into *Cold Shoulders*. Her eyes lit up. Then, I directed her attention to his Left shoulder, which she could see was weighted down because his body leaned that way.

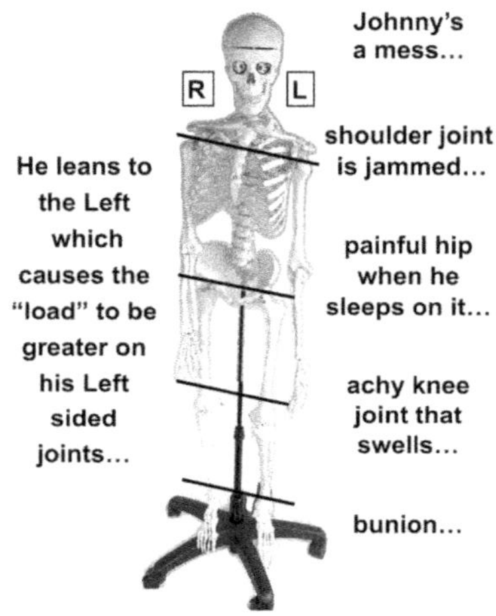

(Image 3C)

Me: *The increased pressure on Johnny's ball and socket has caused his shoulder joint to* ***jam****. When Johnny raises that arm, his shoulder joints rub together, producing an awful grinding sound. It's a mechanically faulty joint that's no longer in its natural alignment, which means it's misaligned.*

At that point, Gabby couldn't contain herself and burst out excitedly.

Gabby: *I want you to look at how I'm standing right now! I definitely have Bowling Ball Head; it's from looking down at my computer all day, right? And it makes perfect sense that it screwed up my shoulder joint. This is amazing... I can't wait for you to show me what I can do to make this better... wait till I tell my mother... she has really bad neck problems and a hump from osteoporosis.*

I quickly glanced at Gabby's side profile while she babbled. Her ear was definitely forward of her shoulder, and her middle-back was pronounced. To make matters worse, I saw a hump and a fat pad. *Oh no,* I said to myself, *Bowling Ball Head, HunchBack Shoulders, and a Dowager's Hump. I believe she'll have more than her fair share of joint problems if she doesn't fix these signs!*

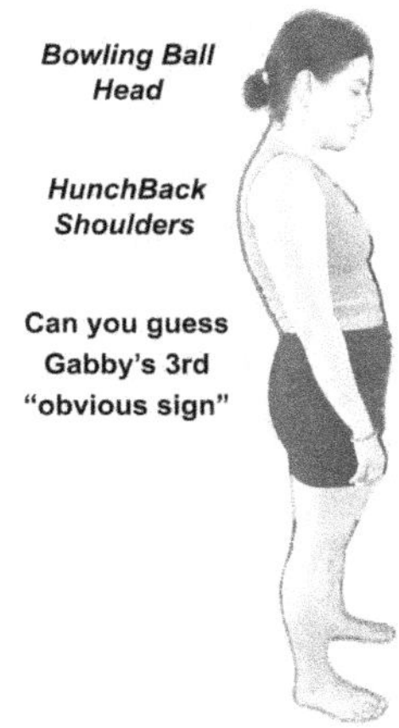

DOWAGER'S HUMP is a condition of the backbone. It is usually associated with *osteoporosis*, but that bone-softening disease doesn't have to be present for a person to develop a lump at the base of their neck. The bony lump develops when neck bones shift forward, and more forward, into an exaggerated *Bowling Ball Head* until neck bone #7 and middle-back bone #1 stick out. A fat pad appears as fat accumulates around the bony lump *(yes, it's actually fat),* which is the body's way of providing additional support to "hold up" the outstretched head. Although I've never heard anyone complain of pain at that site, the skin looks and feels like a puffy pillow.

Johnny's Back-Ender

When the head shifts forward and the shoulders round down, the pelvis has to make a choice… it can push forward into a thrust (like the limbo dance), or it can push backward into a back-ender (so the butt sticks out). See, Johnny's upper body leans forward, his pelvis pushed backward, **and… if… he… had… butt cheeks**, they would be sticking out.

Yes, Johnny's pelvis pushed backward (into a back-ender) after the cement truck rear-ended his car and threw his upper body forward. But a pelvis doesn't NEED the quick force of an accident to be pushed. It can be slowly forced forward into a thrust or slowly forced backward into a back-ender, again and again over its lifetime.

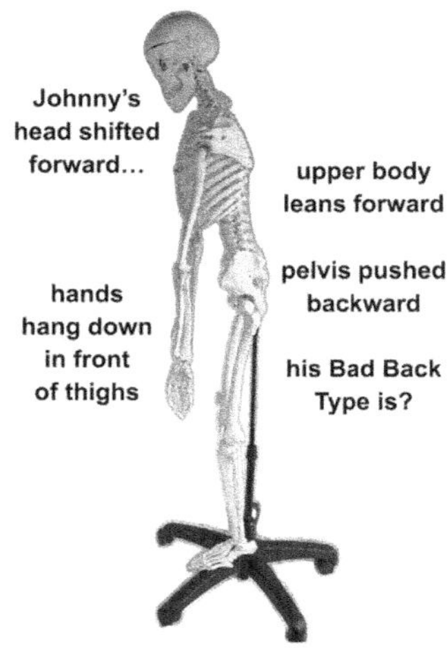

High School Thrust

So, the notion that the pelvis gets **slowly pushed** forward or backward over the course of a lifetime was unexpectedly confirmed as I picked up my tenth grader from high school one afternoon. There I was, about 10 minutes early, parked and waiting just outside the building. With a long line of cars in front of me, I had time to observe the kids mulling about, but it was the kids who huddled together that caught my eye. Backpacks hung off their middle-backs, arms rested over their belly, and their pelvis was pushed **OMG… SO… FAR… FORWARD**. There they were, standing in a pelvic thrust, and ALL I could do was stare disapprovingly…

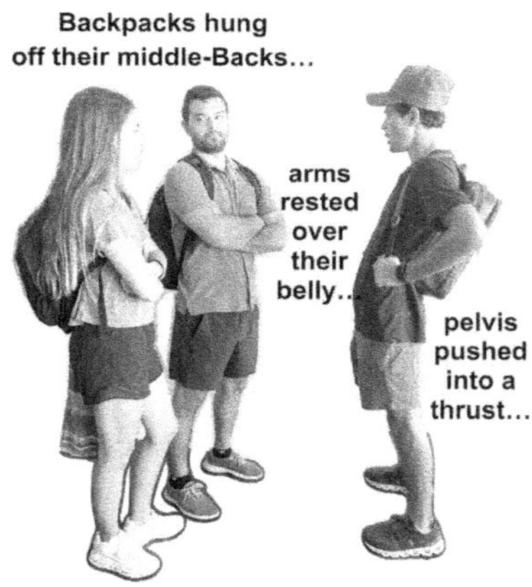

In the next moment, like a flash of lightning, Jeremy opened the door, jumped in, and expected me to high-tail it out of the lineup of cars as if I was his get-away ride. *"Let's go, Mom!"* But MOM wasn't ready. In fact, I did the unthinkable. I asked him to look at the group of kids I was eyeing, desperately wanting to point out this sloppy, slouchy, and awfully suggestive pose. My intentions were to make it clear that he should NEVER be seen standing in a pelvic thrust. As you can imagine, the attempt to educate him was not well received. He chewed me out for "holding up" the line of cars and pointing my finger at his classmates. Apparently, it was the ultimate embarrassment because Jeremy never asked me to pick him up from school again.

That Push Also Rotates

This is known to be true: EVERYBODY'S pelvis will push one way or the other; it just depends on the direction in which it was TRAINED! Like the high school kids who stood around mirroring each other's pelvic thrusts, we **learn** throughout our lifetime to push our pelvis forward into a thrust or backward into a back-ender from the people we "hung out" with the most (parents, siblings, friends). You will continue to reinforce "that push" to accommodate your workstation, a hobby, or because you find it more comfortable. Now, "that push" has become a habit. Unfortunately, the direction in which you trained your pelvis to push doesn't end there.

When you push your pelvis in one direction, it rotates in the opposite direction. This "push and rotate" occurs simultaneously as a single motion. The exercises below will demonstrate this.

Try This —> Stand up and push your pelvis as far forward as possible. *Did you notice your upper body naturally leaned backward?* When the pelvis pushes forward into a thrust, it also rotates backward. That is the 4th Bad Back Sign: *Pelvic Thrust 'n' Tilt.*

Try This —> Stand up and push your pelvis as far backward as possible. *Did you notice your upper body naturally leaned forward?* When the pelvis pushes backward into a back-ender, it also rotates forward. That is the 5th Bad Back Sign: *Pelvic Back-Ender w/ Dip.*

(#4) *PELVIC THRUST 'N' TILT SIGN*

This "sign" occurs when a person's pelvic girdle **pushes forward** (and rotates backward) from its centered alignment. The pelvis is the faulty part of the skeletal structure that influences the sacral base to **tilt backward** and low-back bones to **shift backward** to become the faulty parts of the backbone. This Bad Back Sign is characterized by buttocks that appear "pushed-in."

Quick Glance —> The easiest way to discover if a person has a *Pelvic Thrust 'n' Tilt Sign* is to observe that their upper body leans backward (even slightly), their low-back and buttocks appear straight, and their "backside" clothing hangs straight down.

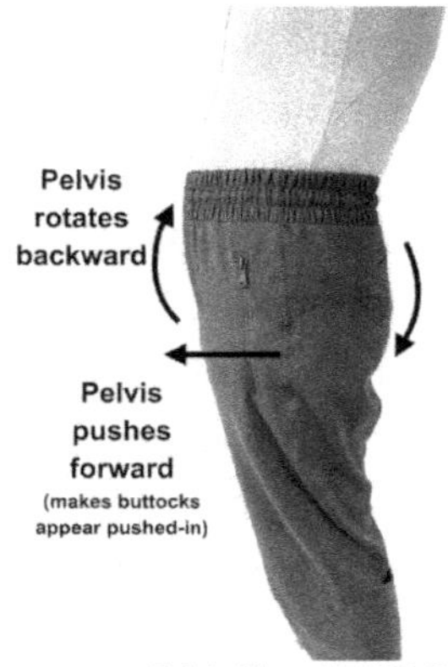

Pelvic Thrust 'n' Tilt Sign

(#5) *PELVIC BACK-ENDER W/ DIP SIGN*

This "sign" occurs when a person's pelvic girdle **pushes backward** (and rotates forward) from its centered alignment. The pelvis is the faulty part of the skeletal structure that influences the sacral base to **dip forward** and low-back bones to **shift forward** to become the faulty parts of the backbone. This Bad Back Sign is characterized by buttocks that appear to be "sticking out."

Quick Glance —> The easiest way to discover if a person has a *Pelvic Back-Ender w/ Dip Sign* is to observe that their upper body leans forward (even slightly), which naturally accentuates their buttocks. This is similar to what a person would look like as they "lean in" to push a stroller or shopping cart.

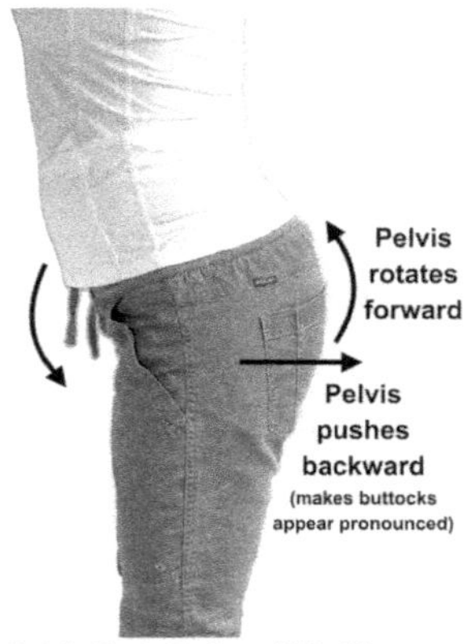

Pelvic Back-Ender w/ Dip Sign

Pelvic Problems Explained

To begin with: it may be helpful to know that the pelvis is NOT part of the backbone; its function is to operate WITH the backbone. Your pelvis, **aka** the pelvic girdle, consists of 2 pelvic bones (ilium) that sandwich the sacrum (the upside-down triangular bone and the 4th curve of the backbone). These 3 large bones give rise to 5 joints; two sacroiliac or SI joints, one L5-S1 sacral base joint, and two femur heads or hip joints.

All 5 joints operate BEST when the pelvis is center-aligned and directly over the ankle. When the pelvis is pushed, the "load" on the 5 articulating joints changes, so it's no longer equally distributed. The joints with the increased "load" become stressed and eventually they jam. Jammed joints become stuck, and stuck joints don't move too well.

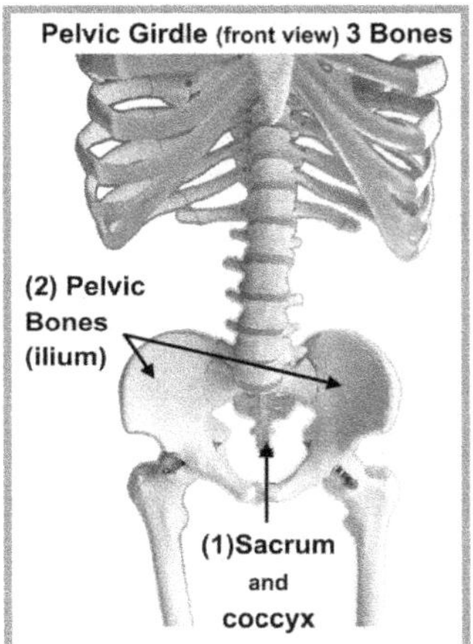

(Image 3D)

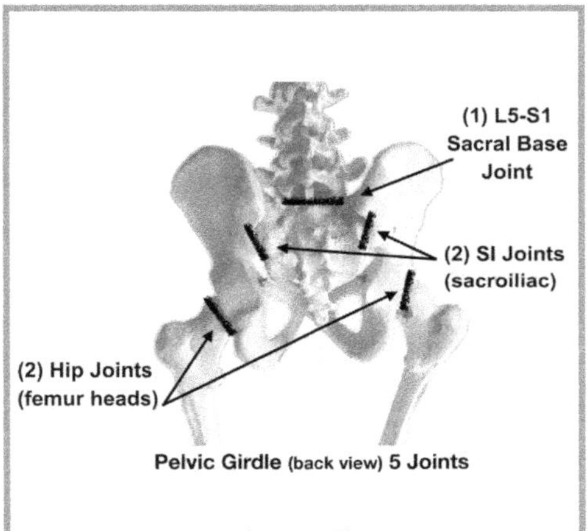

(Image 3E)

SI JOINT DYSFUNCTION is a condition that results when a sacroiliac joint is **jammed** (barely moves) or **stuck** (won't budge). Recall that you have two SI joints, but with this condition, it's usually a one-sided ordeal. Too much "load" on this joint prevents it from moving freely and thriving. However, it's not the only joint of the 5 pelvic joints to **jam**; the L5-S1 (sacral base) joint endures just as much physical stress and pressure. Next time your SI joint inflames and makes it nearly impossible to move in any direction without a muscle spasm and a fair amount of teeth-cringing pain, look to your **pushing pelvis**. Then, go to Step 7 and learn how to reverse your thrust or back-ender to help ALL 5 pelvic joints "share the load."

People Watching

One morning, while out for a run, I caught up to a woman walking her dog. It didn't take me long to notice her walking style. I slowed down to get a better look, and sure enough, I spotted the problem: a pelvic back-ender with a stuck Left SI joint. *Oh boy, was I excited!*

When a person's SI joint is **stuck**, the sacral base (L5-S1 joint) will ALSO stick, which causes a pronounced one-sided, BUTT SWAY. As I studied her butt, I noticed it got pulled to the Right when she extended her Right leg, but when she extended her Left leg, her butt didn't move in that direction**... at all.**

Coupled with her round toosh and pronounced lean forward, I felt proud of myself that I could spot faulty parts and faulty "signs" **on... the... fly!** You, too, can get good at spotting them. Start "people watching" at the grocery store, airport, mall, or wherever you "watch." The more you "watch," the easier it will be to pick out "obvious signs," so keep practicing!

PS: Although this lady had a stuck Left SI joint, I wish I had asked her if she had pain and problems with her Right hip, SI joint, thigh, or knee. I bet she would have said... YES!

STEP 4: LEARN AND OBSERVE THE NOT-SO-OBVIOUS BAD BACK SIGNS

Quirky Head, *Quirky Shoulder*, and *Quirky Pelvis* are the Not-So-Obvious Bad Back Signs that affect the backbone's Vertically Straight Alignment. *Quirky's* are NOT included with the Bad Back Types, but they **can be** identified when you look directly at a person. You might spot one or two, but unlike the "types," *Quirky's* DON'T affect everyone, so it's entirely possible a person has NONE. These stand-alone "signs" don't present themselves in a loud, boisterous way, so a **Quick Glance** doesn't always work; however, your **Structural Evaluation** (Step 6) will reveal whether or not you have any *Quirky's*.

QUIRKY HEAD SIGNS

When a person's head shifts sideways, twists, or tilts from its centered alignment, that's a *Quirky Head Sign*. The head is the faulty part of the skeletal structure that influences neck bones to shift from their Vertically Straight Alignment to become the faulty part of the backbone. The easiest way to discover which direction a person's head has shifted is to observe how their head and neck align with their episternal notch. Facial asymmetry is another clue.

Sideways Head

A sideways head has shifted horizontally Right or Left (use episternal notch as a reference), making the neck appear shortened on the *Quirky* side and stretched on the other.

Try This —> In front of a mirror, shift only your head sideways to the Right (like an Egyptian). This is a Right *Quirky Sideways Head.*

Twisted Head

A twisted head has rotated Right or Left to cause the chin to point toward one shoulder. The ear and face are more visible on the other side.

Try This —> In front of a mirror, rotate your head Left. This is a Left *Quirky Twisted Head.*

Tilted Head

A tilted head bends Right or Left, making the head look diagonally aligned.

Try This —> In front of a mirror, bend your Left ear toward your Left shoulder. This is a Left *Quirky Tilted Head.*

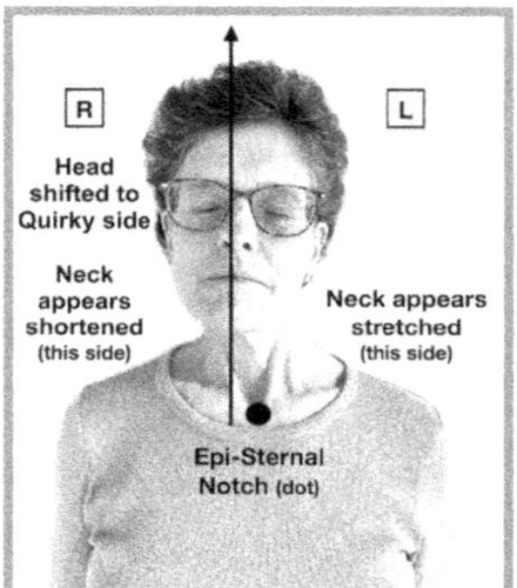

Quirky Sideways Head Sign (Right)

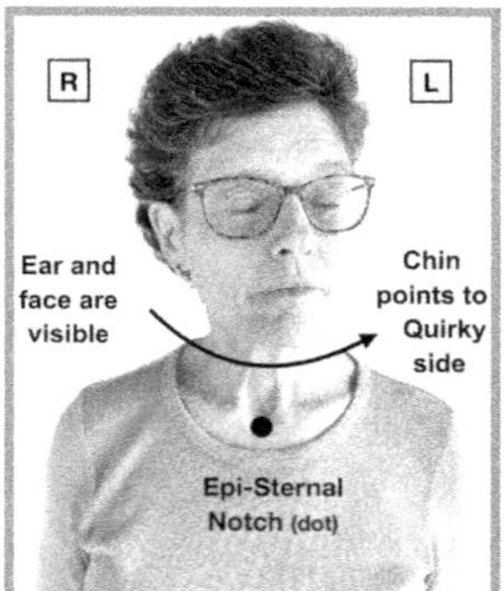

Quirky Twisted Head Sign (Left)

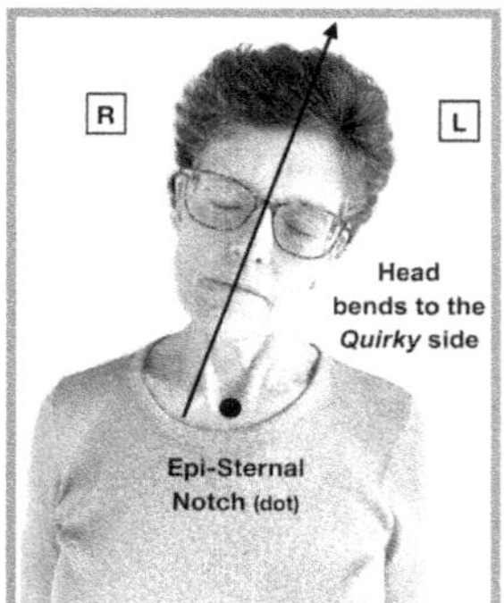

Quirky Tilted Head Sign (Left)

Discussion —> A person with a "head sign" may bend or cock their head (usually to the *Quirky* side) as you talk to them, or you'll notice this in a candid photo. You might see them involuntarily twitch or notice they move their head continuously like they're uncomfortable. These people tend to be clumsy, accident-prone, and often complain they've slept wrong. They may be plagued with an *achy, stiff neck, droopy eyelids, ear, nose,* and *throat problems, fatigue, headaches, grinding teeth, snoring,* and *insomnia.* Additional conditions are possible, such as *dizziness, nausea, vertigo, brain fog, lack of concentration, altered/loss of taste/smell, anxiety, facial palsies, tinnitus,* and other neurological "tics" of the head, neck, and shoulders.

A Goalie's *Quirky Head*

Years ago, I had a case that involved a young ice hockey goalie named AJ, whose poor performance in the net caused him to lose most games for his team. AJ didn't lack goalie skills but struggled to focus on the ice and at school. With teachers pushing to medicate him and a coach ready to replace him, Kathy, his mother, sought another solution and brought him to our office. AJ's **Structural Evaluation** revealed a *Quirky Sideways Head.*

I had only worked with AJ for a couple of months when Kathy excitedly announced that AJ's team had made it to Nationals (because they had twelve straight wins), which secured his "spot" on the team as their STARTING goalie. With tears streaming down her face, Kathy embraced me. "*I cannot thank you enough for helping AJ. After working with you, he said he felt awake, had more energy, and could track the puck better, but more importantly, AJ has settled down at school.*"

Was it a miracle, or because I restored AJ's Quirky Head to its ***centered alignment****? Maybe both!* I accepted Kathy's gratitude and smiled because I had had similar results with other patients.

Quirky Head Signs can be challenging to detect but left uncorrected, problems can persist. This means that whenever the skull, Atlas (neck bone #1), and Axis (neck bone #2) shift sideways, twist, or tilt, they can create a tremendous amount of pressure on the brain stem, which is bound to test the limits of neurological function, just as it did with AJ and the following story.

A Mother Brought To Shame

Speaking of a *Quirky* head reminds me of my son's first concussion. I didn't know what he was experiencing then, but here's how I shamefully handled it.

Jeremy was a hockey player who knew how to cleanly "check" another player (take them out of play). At full speed, his shoulder-to-shoulder contact looked like he was innocently skating past his opponent, but somehow, they'd go flying in another direction. It was during an intense physical game that Jeremy "checked" another player pretty hard. After the game, I waited for him in the car; he opened the back door, slid in, and lay across the seats. *Strange,* I thought. *Jeremy would never sit in the backseat if the front were open... AND... he's lying down!* So I asked, *"Are you okay?"*

"I'm fine, Mom. Let's go."

Jeremy was silent the whole way home, got out of the car, and headed for the couch.

Weird behavior, I thought. I made him a sports drink, and he slept on the couch. When he awoke, I suggested an evaluation, but he rejected the idea, stating he had a headache and wanted to go to bed. I didn't overthink this, but the next morning, I became very concerned when he didn't get up for school.

Hours later, at my insistence, Jeremy dragged himself to the kitchen table and sat with his head buried in his folded arms. Surmising he still had a headache, I asked him what part of his head hurt.

"All over when I move my head, but it goes away when I lay down."

I suddenly felt a sharp pang of guilt in my stomach as the realization hit me; *he had a concussion.* With a serious tone this time, I asked Jeremy to stand up so I could evaluate his head. He stood up, closed his eyes, and slowly lifted his head. I closed my eyes and hung my head in **shame**. It had been twenty hours since his injury, and I had allowed him to rest, which is the protocol for a *concussion, but why, oh why, didn't I adjust him the night before?*

Jeremy's head was severely sideways *(Quirky Sideways Head)*, and his shoulder hung **so** low *(Quirky Shoulder)* that it appeared detached. Immediately, I responded, *"Jeremy, I know you want to go back to bed, but you have to let me shift your head back to the center of your body, or you could remain like this for weeks."*

CONCUSSION is a condition that can occur from a forceful impact to the head that usually elicits an inflammatory response to the organ inside the skull (the brain). Remember, the head sits directly on top of Atlas (neck bone #1), and their joint surfaces rock and roll (Step 3, *Bowling Ball Head*). That means when a force is severe enough to move the skull, Atlas rolls with it, and Axis (neck bone #2) follows. The brain stem travels directly through Atlas and Axis, so when those bones shift, they cause physical stress on the brain stem. As if blowing up like a balloon isn't enough trauma for the brain, the brainstem gets compromised, too. When it comes to *concussions*, ALWAYS check for a *Quirky Head Sign* because the pressure created from a sideways, twisted, or tilted head is bound to elicit some sort of neurological response.

QUIRKY SHOULDER SIGN

When a person's shoulder girdle has shifted from its horizontal alignment, that is a *Quirky Shoulder.* The shoulder is the faulty part of the skeletal structure that influences middle-back bones to shift from their Vertically Straight Alignment to become the faulty part of the backbone. The easiest way to discover this "sign" is to observe a person's shoulders to see if they are level.

Quick Glance —> When you look directly at a person's shoulders, one is HIGHER; that is the *Quirky Shoulder.* You may observe that the thumb on the same side is higher than the other.

Discussion —> A person with this *Quirky* may experience shoulder and middle-back musculoskeletal discomfort and/or dysfunction; *arthritis, bursitis, tendonitis, capsulitis,* or *neuritis.*

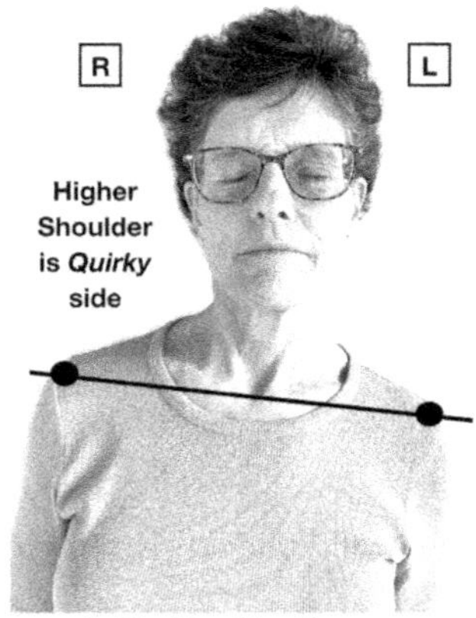

Quirky Shoulder Sign (Right)

QUIRKY PELVIC SIGN

When a person's pelvic girdle shifts sideways from its centered alignment, that is a *Quirky Pelvis.* The pelvis is the faulty part of the skeletal structure that influences the sacrum and low-back bones to shift from their Vertically Straight Alignment to become faulty parts of the backbone. The easiest way to discover this "sign" is to observe a person's pelvis is off to one side, not centered.

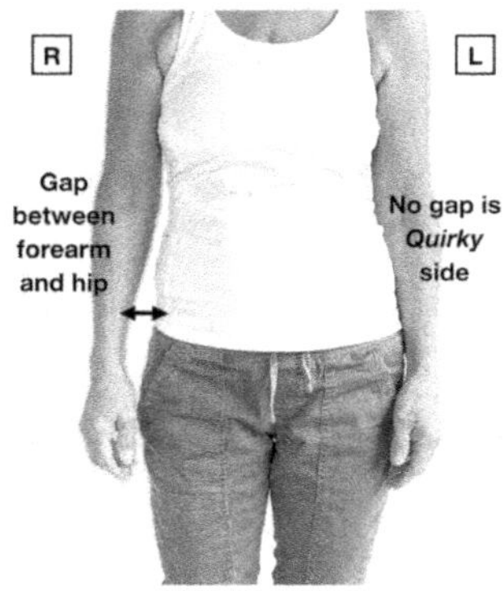

Quirky Pelvic Sign (Left)

Quick Glance —> When you look directly at a person's hips and forearms, you may observe a smaller gap or no gap between hip and forearm; that side is the *Quirky Pelvis.*

Discussion —> A person with this *Quirky* may experience pelvic and low-back musculoskeletal discomfort and/or dysfunction; *arthritis, bursitis, tendonitis, capsulitis, neuritis, discitis, sacroiliitis, or sciatica.*

KNEE AND FOOT PROBLEMS are often the result of a *Quirky Pelvis*. Here's the reason; a pelvis that has shifted sideways will cause body weight to be greater on that side. Inevitably, the "load" gets transferred to the knee and foot, and joint problems are likely. Restore the *Quirky Pelvis* to its natural centered alignment, and like magic, knee and foot issues disappear.

An Active Woman And Her *Quirky Pelvis*

My mother called late one night. Fearing the worst, I picked up the phone to learn that she'd fallen off her porch chair earlier that day and was lying in the hospital waiting for surgery the next morning. I had a hard time believing my very active 75-year-old, health-nut-hippie of a mother could possibly experience a broken bone from a simple fall. As I glanced at the X-ray images she sent via text, sure enough, her femur head was shattered.

Me: *Mom, I know you don't want to hear this, but just because you live six hundred miles away doesn't mean you can't listen to me.*

Mom: *What do you mean, dear daughter?*

Me: *Remember last year when you asked me to check that your Right hip was higher than your Left, but instead, I found your pelvis had shifted sideways to the Right (Right Quirky Pelvis), so it appeared higher. I gave you an orthopedic device to help you re-center it.* I paused. *You've been using it, right?*

Mom: *Faith, to tell you the truth, I forgot all about it, and you live so far away.*

Me: *Mom, femur heads are weight-bearing joints. When your pelvis shifted to the Right, that femur head had to BEAR more load, so it degenerated,* *but when your German Shepherd knocked you off your chair onto the deck, that's the reason it fractured.*

Mom: *Yes, daughter… I should've listened to you.*

STEP 5: DISCOVER THE BAD BACK TYPES

How It All Began

When I opened my first office, I listened to patients complain about their back problems. They'd point to where it hurt, recall details, and then expect me to diagnose EXACTLY *what was wrong*. It wasn't always easy.

As the years passed, I began noticing how faulty **skeletal parts** would repeatedly occur together, so I studied those *parts* with more interest. *Recall*: faulty skeletal parts indicate faulty **backbone parts**. It took me several more years and several hundred patients to gather enough data, confirm my findings, and settle on *three patterns* that consistently occurred together. That's when diagnosing *what was wrong* with a patient's problematic back got much easier and quite exciting! The excitement over this discovery was that a patient could ALWAYS be diagnosed with one of the *three patterns*, no matter how debilitating their symptoms or the clinical name attached to their condition (like *arthritis*, *discitis*, and *sacroiliitis*).

> *That's when it became entirely clear—that pattern—was their back problem!*

Thrilled with the breakthrough, I gave each *pattern* a name, *Front Loader, Boobs Meet Belly,* and *The Stoop*, and referred to them as *Bad Back Syndrome Types*. Identifying a patient's back problem as a "type" made it much easier to communicate **exactly** *what was wrong* with their back. I would say to a new patient, *Tina, your Bad Back Type is Boobs Meet Belly*. We would chuckle, and that was her diagnosis. After reviewing the details of her "type," Tina knew exactly WHERE the problem was, WHICH parts needed to be restored, HOW long it would take, and WHAT she needed to do to take her Bad Back and make it a Good Back.

Why was this the MOST extraordinary "find" of my career? It was a new patient consultation time saver. I no longer needed patients to walk me through all the details, like, WHERE does it hurt? WHEN did it occur? WHAT type of pain? Nor did we waste precious time reviewing HOW their back problems made them miserable, caused them to miss work, or have to postpone social engagements. Instead, we got to focus on something way more productive! We would spend our entire consultation Bad Back "typing" them, then planning what they needed to do to make their Bad Back GOOD again. Not only was this a more efficient use of our time, but it gave the patient hope. *Hope?*

Often, by the time a person ended up in my office, they had already tried many other practitioners and countless treatments, which usually left them feeling like their condition was hopeless. When I began identifying a patient's problem as a Bad Back Type, it made them happy and relieved because, at the end of the day, they just wanted to know *what was wrong* with their back and what they needed to do to get relief.

The "obvious signs," *Bowling Ball Head, Cold Shoulders, HunchBack Shoulders, Pelvic Thrust 'n' Tilt,* and *Pelvic Back-Ender w/ Dip,* are like puzzle pieces from which you will assemble your Bad Back Type. Are you a *Front Loader, Boobs Meet Belly,* or *The Stoop?* Some of you already suspect you have *Bowling Ball Head*, and that's a good start because each "type" is a combination of 3 "obvious signs."

In this step, you will learn about the "types" and how to spot them quickly with **Quick Glance**, and Step 6 will guide you through a **Structural Evaluation** to ensure that you correctly identify your Bad Back Type (and *Quirky's*).

FRONT LOADER (FL) BAD BACK TYPE

You have this "type" if you have these Bad Back Signs: *Bowling Ball Head, Cold Shoulders, Pelvic Thrust 'n' Tilt.*

Quick Glance —> The person with this "type" appears to have *The Good Back Type* as they stand. Upon closer inspection, you'll notice that they lean forward into somewhat of a diagonal alignment or display 1 or 2 definitive "signs" from time to time, which can be confusing. If you can't decipher what "type" a person is, they're probably a *Front Loader.*

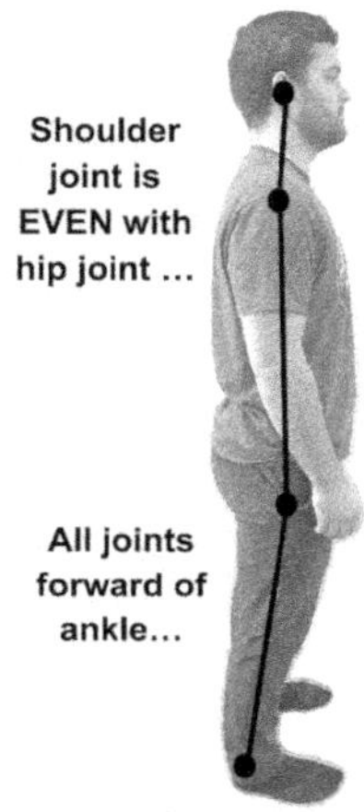

Front Loader Bad Back Type

Discussion —> *Front Loader* is the **initial** "type" to develop. This pattern will **transition** into *Boobs Meet Belly* or *The Stoop* if it isn't reversed. Those with this "type" are usually under the age of fifty, so their joints aren't arthritic or stuck (they could be jammed). That means they can look like either of the other two "types" at any given time. If a person over the age of fifty is "typed" a *Front Loader,* it's usually because they lead an active lifestyle, and their joints are still somewhat flexible. A *Front Loader* may insist that "nothing bothers them" because their complaints are MILD musculoskeletal aches, pains, and problems that they tolerate or eliminate with the help of "over-the-counter" pain medication and exercise.

Josie's *Bunions*

Josie, the HR Director of the company who booked us, sat in the front row during our Lunch 'n' Learn presentation. When I began talking about Johnny's back-ender and asked who would like to know how *bunions* formed, she raised her hand. With Johnny by my side, I pointed to his Left foot to show them his *bunion.* **See page 18, image 2F**. I explained that it formed because his body leaned forward and to the Left, and with the increased load on his Left foot, his arch collapsed, and his big toe was the **last** joint in line to be affected.

Then I stated, *"If your foot has grown in size, a whole size or more, rest assured, you have a collapsed arch."* Josie raised her hand again, but this time with a question. *"You mean to tell me my bunion didn't form as a result of me wearing pointy high-heeled shoes my whole career?"* she asked in a snotty tone.

Another woman quickly raised her hand, wondering if I could help her understand *plantar fasciitis*. *"These are probably two of the most common foot conditions people complain about, and I'm happy to explain the physics behind both. Let's get a volunteer up here so I can show you."*

Kristen, a young woman in her thirties, made her way to the front of the room. I had Kristen stand to make her side profile visible to the audience, then asked her to do the Skeletal Dance. She closed her eyes, shook her head, then marched in place as instructed. The silent audience, anxious to see how her physique would change, waited patiently. Kristen was of average height and weight, and when her athletic body finally stood still, we could see that she appeared to be standing fairly straight. I asked the audience if Kristen's ear was in line with her shoulder.

Audience: *No, it's in front.*

Me: *Good, that means she's got Bowling Ball Head... Is Kristen's shoulder in line with her hip joint?*

Audience: *Yes.*

Me: *Is Kristen's hip in line with her ankle joint?*

Audience: *No, it's in front.*

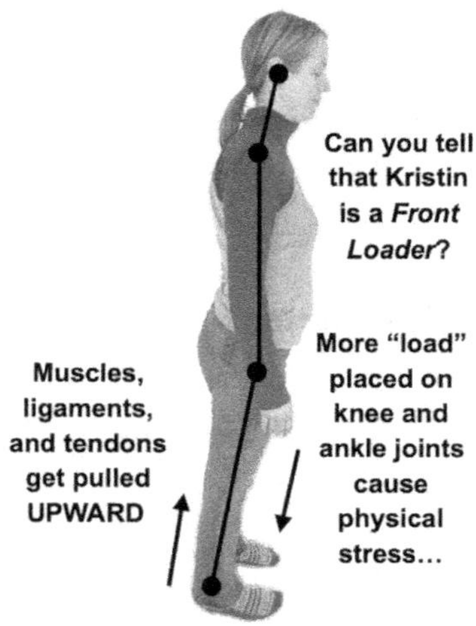

(Image 5A)

Me: *Okay, let's confirm; Kristen's ear, shoulder, and hip are forward of her ankle, so she appears diagonally aligned. That presentation makes her Bad Back Type, Front Loader.*

I quietly asked Kristen if she had any knee or foot problems that she was comfortable sharing with the audience.

Kristen: *I have shin splints.*

Me: *Great! I mean, I'm not glad you have shin splints, but you've just helped me prove my point.*

My Point

When a person's body hangs over their ankles, their knees and feet joints bear the brunt of their weight. Eventually, conditions like *shin splints, bunions,* and *plantar fasciitis* can develop. Most would never consider how the physics of their skeletal structure changed to create those conditions. If you are a *Front Loader* and don't have any problems yet, I urge you to take your mild "signs" seriously!

> ***SHIN SPLINTS*** are a condition that develops when more load/pressure is placed on the anterior knee and ankle joints. This physical stress **shoves** attached muscles, ligaments, and tendon fibers together, which shortens and tightens them. The soft tissue will cramp when an "activity" stresses them.

> ***BUNIONS*** are a condition that's more apt to form if the afflicted has worn tight, narrow, and pointy high-heeled shoes for many years. However, the problem is that **any size heel** (higher than the footbed) will push the body forward, so the balls of the foot receive more "load" than the heels. Over time, this increased stress causes the arches to collapse, which increases the pressure on the big toe, and eventually, the "bunion joint" shifts off to the side.

PLANTAR FASCIITIS is a condition that develops when the pelvis pushes either forward or backward and the muscles, ligaments, and tendons get **pulled upward** from the bottom of the foot up the back of the leg (calf muscle). In other words, the soft tissue is continually stretched when a person stands, walks, and jogs. The tired and weakened muscles grow weary and fatigue, then spasm, and *voilà*, *plantar fasciitis* or other conditions like a *pulled hamstring, a torn calf muscle,* or *Achilles tendonitis* could result. If you are wearing a nighttime brace to deal with this condition, consider reversing your pelvic "sign" and check out Foot Therapy, Step 9.

A Balancing Act

When the head shifts forward and the shoulders round down, the pelvis **will** make a choice... it **will** push backward until the butt sticks out... or it **will** push forward until the boobs sit on the belly! The latter was fairly common with the older population that came to our office, and I used to refer to it as *old man posture* until I had an *"aha"* moment. It happened during one of my Lunch 'n' Learns.

There I was, standing in the middle of the room surrounded by 30, 40, and 50-year-olds, demonstrating *old man posture.* I jutted my head forward, rounded my shoulders, and "sat" on my middle-back. Then, with all the pelvic flexibility I could muster, I pushed my pelvis as far forward as it would go. I paused for a second, and that's when it hit me; *my boobs just got closer to my belly.* So I blurted out, "*This is what could happen to you in your elder years if you don't fix the **bad** parts of your back—your BOOBS will meet your BELLY!"* The audience erupted in laughter, and the name stuck.

Boobs Meet Belly Bad Back Type is the perfect example of a balancing act. As humans, we've been equipped with a balancing mechanism that self-adjusts our body in an effort to keep us upright so we don't fall flat on our faces when we stand. This is how the *Boobs Meet Belly* "balancing act" works.

- The more the head and neck bones shift forward (*Bowling Ball Head)*...
- The more the middle-back bones shift backward (*HunchBack Shoulders*)...
- The more the pelvis pushes forward (*Pelvic Thrust 'n' Tilt*)...

It's a "balancing act" that's sure to bring whatever size boobies you have **closer** to whatever size belly you have...

BOOBS MEET BELLY (BMB) BAD BACK TYPE

You have this "type" if you have these Bad Back Signs: *Bowling Ball Head, HunchBack Shoulders, Pelvic Thrust 'n' Tilt.*

Quick Glance —> The person with this "type" can be observed standing, like in conversation, with their head and pelvis pushed forward while they "sit" back on their middle-back and often cross their arms above their belly. This appearance ranges from *noticeable* to *no question about it,* but if they have a FLAT BUTT, it's a dead giveaway.

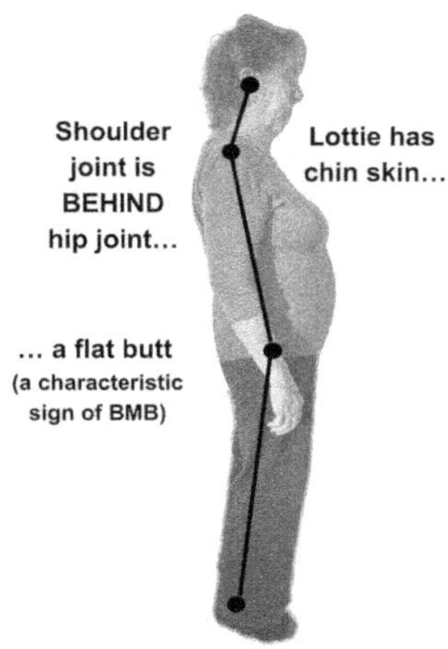

Boobs Meet Belly Bad Back Type

(Image 5B)

Discussion —> If the skeletal structure of a *Front Loader* is allowed to degrade, it will **transition** into *Boobs Meet Belly.* This "type" is the easiest to pick out because of its unmistakable "balancing act" appearance. In an **early stage**, a person may have mild to moderate musculoskeletal aches, pains, and problems. See Step 3, Gabby has this "type." The **advanced stage** is characterized by drastic shifts of the head and pelvis, and they often stand with knees bent. See Step 1, Lou has this "type." By the time someone reaches this stage, they have moderate to severe physical dysfunction, which is often greater than their discomfort.

Have You Shrunk

If a young person (in their 20s or 30s) made an appointment with our office, it was usually because they had attended one of our Lunch 'n' Learns. Motivated to take their mild neck and low-back discomfort seriously, they'd announce, *"I'm here because I don't want to look like my grandmother or grandfather."*

This reminds me of a presentation I gave at a senior center. It happened when I was demonstrating *Boobs Meet Belly* that an older gentleman got up from his seat and shuffled to the front of the room where I was standing with Johnny Bones. Since I didn't ask for a volunteer, I was confused. Without a word, he reached out and touched Johnny's backbone. Sliding his hand from the top of Johnny's neck to his middle-back, the man looked at me and asked, *"Could this be why I've lost two inches?"*

Relieved, I took a deep breath and, with a comforting softness in my voice, directed my answer to the audience. *"It can take decades for the skeletal structure to degrade into an **advanced stage**, and along the way, it **will** alter height. I will teach you today how to restore your backbone's strength, stability, and springy-ness, and as a side benefit, some of the height you've lost will be regained."* I had just barely finished speaking when a woman from the audience shouted, *"Well, let's get on with it!"*

I guess I was a little surprised to be heckled by a group of seniors, and as I glanced over to see who made the comment, I was inspired by the women's appearance to discuss something I don't often get the chance to talk about. I quickly replied, *"I have something you will be thrilled to learn about before I teach you how to lift your boobs off your belly. Would anyone like to know about chin skin?"* I lifted my chin, grabbed my throat skin, and pulled it out as I spoke. And as if I didn't already have these people's attention, they sat upright in their chairs and opened their eyes a little wider.

Naturally, I wanted to evaluate my heckler's structure for the crowd, so I invited her onstage. Lottie stood maybe five feet tall and had more going on than just her boobs resting on her stomach; Lottie had *chin skin* and a characteristic sign indicative of *Boobs Meet Belly*... a flat butt!

CHIN SKIN is a condition that develops when the head shifts forward into an **exaggerated** *Bowling Ball Head.* It can cause the neck curve to straighten and the throat skin to stretch. With gravity's help, the skin begins to sag, and it may take years to become flabby, but when it does, *chin skin* looks an awful lot like the red waddle hanging from a chicken's beak.

FLAT BUTTS are a characteristic sign of the Pelvic Thrust 'n' Tilt. It develops as the pelvis rotates backward, and the sacral base TILTS backward, which causes its "pointy end" (coccyx) to TUCK inward, like a tail between the legs. This "sacral tuck" is what causes the butt to "flatten" and the low-back Master Curve to straighten for a "lack of definition" appearance (see Lou, Step 1). Wanna "beef up" a flat butt? It is possible; you must reverse your pelvic tilt and put a good amount of effort into the Walking Habit (Step 9).

SCIATICA is a condition that causes annoying, painful (sometimes debilitating), radiating symptoms that travel down the butt, thigh, and leg. Plagued with this condition, patients would tell me, *"The throbbing pain down my leg as I drive is SO BAD, I just want to cut my leg off!"* The sciatic nerve is formed as low-back nerve roots (L1-L5) unite into a large single nerve that passes deep within the butt muscles to continue down the leg. **See page 23, image 2G**. You have a Left and Right sciatic nerve, but if you suffer from *sciatica*, you've probably experienced irritation on only one side (often the result of a *Quirky Pelvis*). When a person's skeletal structure transitions into *Boobs Meet Belly*, it's like a *tug-of-war*; *Bowling Ball Head* pulls the spinal cord (encased inside the backbone) from the **top** of the backbone and *Thrust 'n' Tilt* pulls the spinal cord from the bottom. Remember, nerve roots attach to the spinal cord, and DON'T like to be pinched (compressed) or pulled (stretched). *Sciatica* occurs when low-back spinal nerve roots (L1- L5) are compressed and stretched, which causes them to produce a variety of neurological symptoms such as: sharp, stabbing, burning, throbbing, and/or radiating signals, pins/needles, temperature changes, and/or muscle weakness… all the way down the leg. With every case of *sciatica* that "presented" to our office, the sufferer always had *Boobs Meet Belly*. The more exaggerated their *Bowling Ball Head*, the greater the symptoms.

CERVICAL RADICULOPATHY is a condition that causes annoying, painful (sometimes debilitating), radiating symptoms that travel down the arm, forearm, and sometimes into the hand. When a person's skeletal structure transitions into *Boobs Meet Belly*, it's like a *tug-of-war*; *Bowling Ball Head* pulls the spinal cord (encased inside the backbone) from the **top** of the backbone and *Thrust 'n' Tilt* pulls the spinal cord from the bottom. Again, nerve roots attach to the spinal cord, and don't like to be pinched (compressed) or pulled (stretched). *Cervical Radiculopathy* occurs when neck spinal nerve roots (C1-C8) are compressed and stretched which causes them to produce a variety of neurological symptoms such as: sharp, stabbing, burning, throbbing, and/or radiating signals, pins/needles, temperature changes, and/or muscle weakness... all the way down the arm. With every case of *cervical radiculopathy* that "presented" to our office, the sufferer always had *Boobs Meet Belly*. The more exaggerated their *Bowling Ball Head*, the greater the symptoms.

The Push Determines The Type

When the head shifts forward and the shoulders round down, the pelvis will make a choice… it **will** push forward until the boobs sit on the belly… or it **will** push backward until the butt sticks out, and *The Stoop* takes form. *The Stoop* also develops from *Front Loader*, but only after the pelvis is pushed, pushed, and continually pushed backward throughout one's lifetime.

THE STOOP (ST) BAD BACK TYPE

You have this "type" if you have these Bad Back Signs: *Bowling Ball Head, Cold Shoulders, Pelvic Back-Ender w/ Dip.*

Quick Glance —> The person with this "type" can be observed standing with their upper body leaning forward over their waist. If it's just a smidgen, you'll have to glance harder. If the lean is drastic, they will appear "stooped over." A small round butt is telltale, but a BIG round BUTT is a dead giveaway.

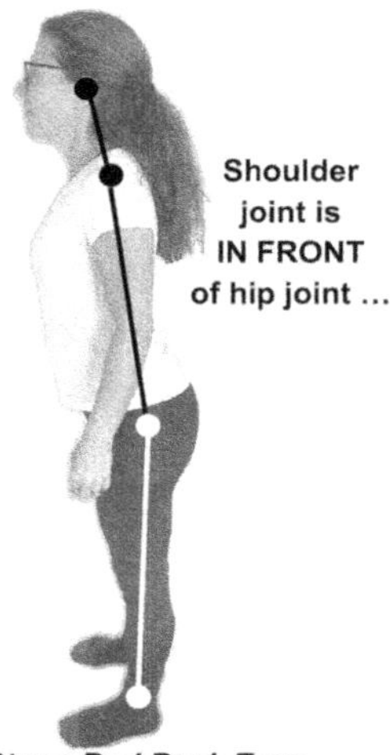

The Stoop Bad Back Type

Discussion —> If the skeletal structure of a *Front Loader* is allowed to degrade, it will **transition** into *The Stoop*. The person with this "type" leans forward while standing, walking, and running. They also lean on a counter or furniture with their butt pushed backward. In an **early stage**, individuals have mild to moderate musculoskeletal aches, pains, and problems, especially with forward bending activities (vacuuming, gardening, washing dishes). A person in an **advanced stage** may struggle to walk without the assistance of a cane or walker. By the time they reach this stage, they have moderate to severe physical dysfunction, which is often greater than their discomfort. See Step 3, Johnny Bones has this "type."

Erin's *Stoop* Was Irish

Megan walked in, excited to announce, *"I've got my best friend Erin in the car. She's in a lot of pain and can't stand up or walk very well. I've been talking about you for years, and now that she's in a pretty bad way, she's finally agreed to see you."*

The entire office stared at Erin as she walked in with Megan's assistance. Immediately, I saw the problem. Erin's exaggerated lean and pronounced back-ender gave it away, but then her red hair, thin torso, and hefty thighs told me her *Stoop* was definitely Irish. I hadn't seen this exaggerated posture since my trip to Ireland in the nineties, but Erin's *Stoop* took the prize with her upper body literally folded in half at her waist so she could barely look straight ahead. Erin's major complaint was that she couldn't stand for any length of time before her low-back would go into a spasm and shoot pain in every direction. To make matters worse, Erin was uncomfortable in any position but sitting, which didn't work too well for her with two small children at home. Why she waited so long to do something about her condition didn't make sense to any of us.

When I asked Erin how long she'd been stooped over, she responded, *"All my life, I don't ever remember standing up straight. I grew up picking potatoes on my parents' farm back home in Ireland, and when you meet them, you'll see we all look the same. Now that I think about it, my Mom suffers from gripping back pain just like me, and my dad already had two back surgeries!"*

This scenario may cause you to wonder, *"Are Bad Back Types inherited or learned?"* Often, a parent and child would "present" to our office with the same Bad Back Type and the same low-back or neck complaints. It makes sense; they sit on the same couch, lean on the same table, and mirror each other's standing gestures and behaviors. When Erin came to our office, her *Stoop* was already advanced, which was atypical for her age, so she likely inherited the skeletal weakness and trained her structure to resemble her parents every time she sat, stood, and walked.

LOW BACK NERVE COMPRESSION is a condition that occurs when low-back bones shift out of their Master Curve (tend to straighten) to compress and stretch the L1-L5 spinal nerve roots. Remember, nerve roots DON'T like to be pinched or pulled. Nerves that experience tension often respond with burning and throbbing sensations, and sometimes pain can radiate down a leg or stay localized and **shoot** pain in every direction.

BULGING AND HERNIATED DISCS are conditions that commonly occur when the pelvis pushes into a thrust or back-ender, and the low-back Master Curve is compromised. The process of going from a curve to straight is an All-Shift-Together Misalignment that forces the bones to jam, and that is where the problem begins. When bones are shoved together, nerve roots are likely to become pinched and pulled, which causes them to produce sharp, stabbing, and radiating symptoms. It's possible the **jammed** bones squish the disc outward like cheese **oozing** out the sides of your grilled cheese sandwich. With *Boobs Meet Belly*, disc problems usually occur at L4-L5 and/or L5-S1. With *The Stoop*, disc problems usually occur at L1-L2 and/or L2-L3. The difference in location is likely caused by joints that had to "bear more load" as a person assumed either "type." Bulging discs usually develop with a slow force, whereas herniations usually develop with a quick force.

Don't Wait

With "signs" and "types" dancing around in your head, *you might be questioning whether your stiff back, grinding neck bones, achy shoulders, or tingling toes are purely the fault of your skeletal structure.* Yes, remember, *Bad Back Syndrome* comes first. All muscle, nerve, joint, or disc problems occur secondary and therefore should **ALWAYS** be blamed on one's *Bad Back Syndrome **Type**.* Simply put, you are either a *Front Loader, Boobs Meet Belly,* or *The Stoop*. That is the problem, regardless of your pain and dysfunction or no pain and function.

Don't wait to address your outstretched head, rounded shoulders, or flat butt. You might not be folded in half yet, but those "signs," even in the early stage, indicate current or future problems. With the help of a **Structural Evaluation**, you will correctly identify your Bad Back Type, and Step 7 will teach you how to reverse it.

STEP 6: DETERMINE YOUR BAD BACK TYPE AND A QUIRKY OR TWO

On The Road

Before I retired from clinical practice to write this book, I took *The Bad Back To Good Back Program* on the road to a drug and alcohol recovery center. Our program's purpose was to offer physical support to substance abuse clients by improving their Bad Back Signs. Our motto was *"look good and feel good."*

At the center, a client's recovery plan usually involved thirty days of standard medical treatment, and our program ran concurrently. Over the course of a client's stay, I worked with them weekly. The following stories are a couple of my favorite cases.

Jai's Story

Jai was a sturdy and "wired" cowgirl who talked decibels above a normal conversation level and, with a high-pitched twang, made her presence known. I loved her the moment she walked through the door as I watched her make her way through a group of clients to sit properly on my adjusting table, ready and willing to talk. This was the opposite of how most clients "presented" themselves.

She announced, *"I've been to many practitioners over the years, and I still have an ache around my Left shoulder blade that occasionally pinches me, and I'm always dropping things because my hand doesn't seem to have the same strength as it used to. A while back, someone said it was probably scoliosis. Wanna see my bump?"*

She whipped off her hoodie and bent at the waist, so her Left shoulder blade visibly flared. Tender to the touch and downright painful when poked, her condition resulted in a fair amount of muscle weakness that extended from her shoulder to her hand as I performed muscle and neurological tests. I used my tablet (to take a picture) for Jai's **Structural Evaluation**, which made it easy to see her Bad Back Signs. Jai anxiously waited for me to print her a copy of the photo and gasped when she saw her head was indeed shifted forward *(Bowling Ball Head)* and shifted Left *(Quirky Sideways Head).* Fascinated to see her Bad Back Type was *Front Loader,* I gave her the picture and explained the essence of my program was to improve her "signs" with weekly adjustments and molding stretches that she could do at the center and continue when she returned home.

"You're gonna screw my head back on straight?" she asked with a giggle. "*Cause that's exactly what I think I need, and by golly, I'm ready!"*

See what I'm talking about? Who wouldn't love to help this girl? Bound and determined to see and feel the results I assured her were possible, I saw Jai ten times over the course of her thirty-day program. We saw a nice improvement when we compared her *before and after* pictures, and this is what she wrote in her testimonial:

> *"I've had backbone care before, but not like this. Your program is so effective, and I no longer have that annoying shoulder problem or jaw pain. You've taught me so much about what I can do to keep my head on top of my shoulders, and I will keep up the stretches when I go home because I can eat steak now without jaw pain! Thank you; you're amazing!"*

Jai never mentioned that she had *TMJ*, but hearing that it was resolved made me feel good. Additionally, Jai shared that she would live with her parents and finish her degree instead of going back to work on the ranch. She wore a big smile as we talked, and I sensed her confidence in her new plan.

TMJ is a condition involving two jaw joints: the temporal and the mandibular. Those with this problem will tell you it's downright painful to open their mouth fully, and they avoid eating foods that require chewing and grinding. The problem with the temporal-mandibular joints is that they are **misaligned**. Blame it on a *Quirky Sideways, Twisted, or Tilted Head* that placed more load on **one** of the mandibular joints until it **jammed**. Despite rubbing and clicking, the sufferer continues eating, so the nerves inflame, and the muscles spasm. I've helped many *TMJ* cases, and they all had a *Quirky Bowling Ball Head* in common. When those "signs" were reversed, the patient could eat normally again. If you wear a nighttime mouth guard to deal with this condition, consider reversing your *Quirky Head* "signs."

SUPRASCAPULAR NERVE PALSY is a nerve-related condition characterized by annoying neck and shoulder pain. Symptoms include muscle weakness that makes holding a cup of coffee or raising the hands above the head challenging. The suprascapular nerve (sends energy to the shoulder blade) branches from spinal nerve roots sandwiched between neck bones C5, 6, 7, and T1. Unfortunately, a straightened neck curve will pinch or pull those spinal nerve roots and compromise nerve energy coming and going to the suprascapular nerve. Without sufficient nerve energy, muscles don't get vital nutrients, and slowly, they weaken and waste away. Those with upper back curvatures (*scoliosis*) are prone to this condition. **See page 96, image 7B.**

Doug's Story

Doug was anything but chatty. With a solemn expression on his face and his head hung low, he stumbled over to meet me, mostly out of curiosity, he admitted. It took him over two weeks and lots of prodding by a good handful of clients who urged him to *see Dr. Faith because she would make him feel better.*

Some clients needed a week or more of detoxing before they could think clearly enough to make it to my clinic. Doug was one of those cases. He didn't say much, left his intake form blank, and mumbled; *nothing bothered him.* I briefly glanced at his paperwork, flashed him a smile, and felt a pang in my heart. Intuitively, I knew Doug would do well with our program.

After Doug's **Structural Evaluation**, I showed him the printout so he could see he was a *Front Loader.* Then I explained that if he followed through with my recommendations, he would stand tall and look as handsome as ever. Doug looked at me and, without any expression, responded, "*Okay, what do I need to do?*"

Doug rarely missed a session with me over the course of his two-month stay, and within a few weeks, his ho-hum attitude became noticeably cheerful and engaging. His appearance went from shabby to clean-cut, and he had *more energy than he'd ever had* (his exact words). I had noticed something else about Doug; he no longer stumbled over his words but was clear with his thought process and communication. Whereas before, I might have described Doug as emotionally unavailable, he was now fully present and alert. **See page 160, image 10A**.

As I reflect on our work at the recovery center, I can say without hesitation that *The Bad Back To Good Back Program* was successful. I owe that success entirely to the **Structural Evaluation.** *Here's why:* physical improvements and other positive changes can follow when Bad Back Signs are correctly identified and reversed. The clients we worked with would agree.

The Key To Determining Your Bad Back Type

When a person's structure is evaluated, **faulty skeletal parts** (head, shoulders, pelvis) reveal themselves as Bad Back Signs and *Quirky's*. Those "signs" indicate **faulty backbone parts** (neck, middle-back, low-back, sacrum), which are the problem parts. When you evaluate your structure… you **correctly identify** your Bad Back Signs and *Quirky's*. Those "signs" ARE your problem parts, the ROOT cause of your back problems, and the **KEY** to determining your Bad Back Type.

STRUCTURAL EVALUATION ACTIONS 1-5

To determine your Bad Back Type, follow ALL 5 Actions:

Action #1 – Recall *The Good Back Type*
Action #2 – Prepare Space And Subject
Action #3 – Do Skeletal Dance
Action #4 – Take Pictures
Action #5 – Complete/Interpret Structural Evaluation

ACTION #1—RECALL THE GOOD BACK TYPE

From the top of your head to the bottom of your feet, until you die, you SHOULD be standing in *The Good Back Type*. **See page 10, images 1A, 1B, 1C, 1D**. Remember, at the end of Step 1, we briefly discussed that *The Good Back Type* is the natural (not forced) standing alignment of a person's skeletal parts. Let's jog your memory.

The Good Back Side View Alignment

Your ear, shoulder, hip, knee, and ankle joints should line up. When those skeletal parts NATURALLY line up (without you forcing them), it's a good indication that your backbone parts (neck, middle-back, low-back, sacrum) have a 4 Curve Alignment, and you have *The Good Back Type*. If those **skeletal parts** DON'T line up, **you've got** *Front Loader, Boobs Meet Belly,* or *The Stoop* Bad Back Type.

The Good Back Front View Alignment

Your head (and chin) should line up with your episternal notch (bony groove under the throat). Your shoulders should be horizontally level, and your pelvis center-aligned. When those skeletal parts NATURALLY line up (without you forcing them), it's a good indication that your backbone parts have a Vertically Straight Alignment, and you DON'T have *Quirky's*. If those **skeletal parts** DON'T line up, **you've got** *Quirky's.*

Marcie's Evaluation

Marcie jumped out of her seat when I asked for a volunteer. Excited to be evaluated, she ran up on stage, ditched her shoes, and waited for my direction. I instructed Marcie to close her eyes, shake her head, march in place, and relax her body (the skeletal dance).

I explained to the audience that when Marcie closed her eyes, her brain would turn OFF its balancing mechanism to reveal her body's true imbalances (skeletal parts that don't line up). While I was speaking, Marcie's physique slowly but surely changed. I asked the audience to look at her side profile to see if Marcie's ear was in line with her shoulder. Then, I stepped to the back of the room for a better view. *Wow!* I thought to myself. *I couldn't have asked for a better candidate!* Then someone shouted, *"Marcie's got Bowling Ball Head."*

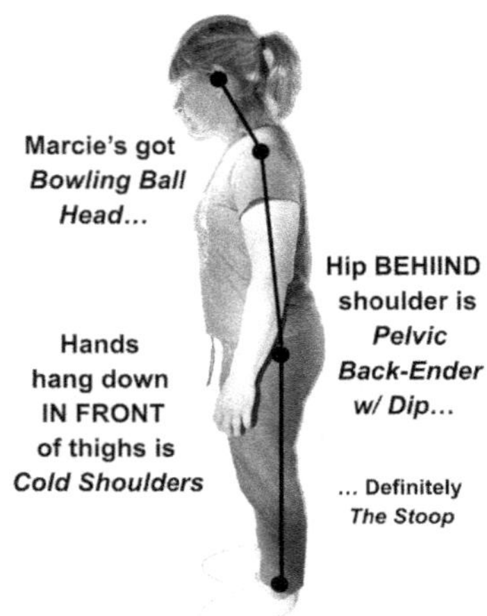

Me: *Yep, Marcie's ear is definitely in front of her shoulder. Is her shoulder in line with her hip joint?*

Audience: *No.*

Me: *Ok, when the hip is found behind the shoulder, it's the Pelvic Back-Ender* *w/ Dip Sign, and it causes the hands to fall out in front of the thighs. Can anyone remember the name of that sign?*

The audience was silent, so I fixed myself behind Marcie and gently pulled her upper body and shoulders backward until her hands landed alongside her thighs. I said, *This is where the hands should naturally hang, which means Marcie has Cold Shoulders and definitely has The Stoop.*

ACTION #2—PREPARE SPACE AND SUBJECT

The **subject** is the person being evaluated. **Subject**, follow these instructions:

- For the evaluation to be most successful, use a well-lit space in front of a blank wall.
- Clothes should be tight-fitting. Wear a tank top or a sleeveless shirt so the **shoulder joints** and episternal **notch** are visible. The hip, knee, and ankle joints are best seen when wearing shorts or leggings. If wearing jeans, use the rivet to gauge where the hip joint is located. Roll the Left pant leg up so the **knee** and **ankle joints** are visible.
- Take socks and shoes off, and tie the hair back so the **ear** is visible.
- Stand with ONLY your Right shoulder facing the wall (don't lean against it), feet hip-width apart, and feet horizontally level.

ACTION #3—DO SKELETAL DANCE

The Skeletal Dance will reveal how the **subject's** skeletal parts line up. **Subject**, follow these "dance" instructions:

- Close your eyes. Shake your head up and down (3x) and side to side (3x), then position your head straight ahead but keep your eyes closed. Next, march in place (3x), then relax your body completely.
- Be calm, and DO NOT force your body into *The Good Back Type* because that would **defeat the purpose**. It will take 30 seconds

for your skeletal structure to "reveal" its faulty alignment and 60 seconds for the **observer** to take two pictures.

Skeletal Dance Mirror-Mirror-Method

You can do the Skeletal Dance in front of a mirror if you would like to evaluate yourself (without the help of an **observer**). This Mirror-Mirror-Method won't give you a picture, and it only works for the front view, but it's quite effective for spotting *Quirky's*. Use a full-length mirror to evaluate your whole body or a bathroom mirror to evaluate just your head and shoulders. The challenge with this method is that after you "do the dance" and wait 30 seconds to open your eyes to start the evaluation, your brain starts to balance you almost immediately. So, if you decide to use this method, you'll have to act very quickly. I recommend repeated attempts until you can determine whether or not you have any *Quirky's*.

Disrupt Brain Equilibrium

The reasoning behind the Skeletal Dance is to intentionally disrupt the brain's equilibrium. The eyes feed the brain information, so when they're open, the brain tries to hold the body in balance. When the eyes are closed, the brain releases "its hold" to "reveal" the skeletal structure's true imbalances.

ACTION #4—TAKE PICTURES

The **observer** is the person taking pictures of the **subject**. **Observer**, follow these instructions:

- Grab a phone or tablet.
- Ensure there's sufficient distance between you and the **subject** to take one side view and one front view, head-to-toe picture. Kneel to get a straight-on, middle-body view.
- Ask the **subject** to "do the dance" (shake, march, relax).

- Wait 30 seconds after the **subject** has "danced," so their Bad Back Signs have time to "reveal" themselves. Take the side-view picture NOW.
- Ask the **subject** to open their eyes, do a half-turn TO FACE YOU, and check that their feet are horizontally level. Ask the **subject** to close their eyes and "do the dance" again. Wait 30 seconds so their *Quirky's* have time to "reveal" themselves. Take the front-view picture NOW.

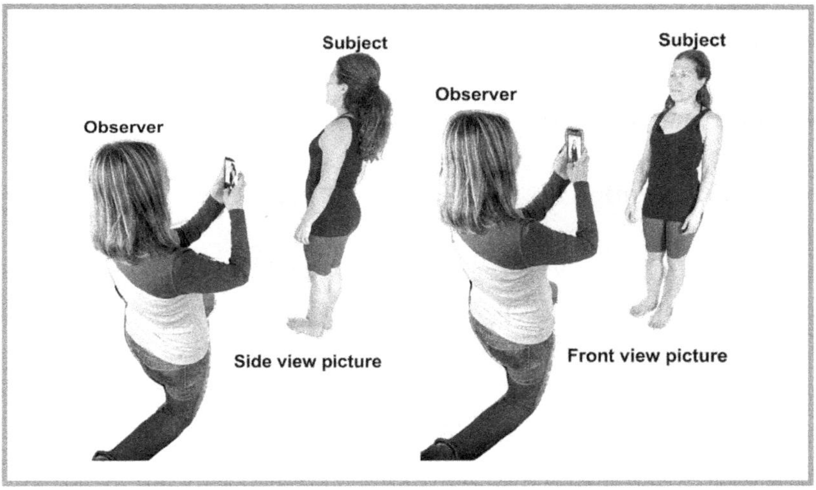

You Only Need Eyeballs

Back at the office, for new patients, I used to rely solely on their Structural Evaluation and plain film X-rays to give me ALL necessary information. I took X-rays because they are the ONLY way to accurately measure the backbone's Vertically Straight and 4 Curve Alignment (to reveal misalignments). The reason I evaluated a patient's skeletal structure was equally simplistic; it revealed faulty skeletal parts, which indicate faulty backbone parts (misalignments). With both diagnostic tests giving me the same information, I confidently knew WHAT parts were the patient's problem parts.

When I was at the recovery center, the ONLY diagnostic test I had available was a client's **Structural Evaluation,** but that single test proved highly effective. Take Jai's evaluation for instance; her head was shifted forward and sideways to give her a *Quirky Bowling Ball Head.* A sideways head indicates neck bones have a compromised Vertically Straight Alignment. A forward head indicates a compromised Master Curve. Just by visually examining her structure, I was able to identify Jai's problem parts, which were likely the cause of her *TMJ* and *suprascapular neuritis.*

A Structural Evaluation is highly effective, so much so that you ONLY need your eyeballs, the pictures you just took, and Action #5.

ACTION #5—COMPLETE/INTERPRET STRUCTURAL EVALUATION

PART I: Determine the Subject's Bad Back Type

To begin, use the subject's side view picture and the Side View Structural Evaluation Chart (to print the chart, go to our website). Follow the observation instructions given on the chart. For additional guidance, refer to the Bad Back Signs detailed in Step 3 and *The Good Back Type* pictures. **See page 10, images 1A, 1C**. This part will be easier to complete if you **expand** the subject's picture on the phone or tablet. To assess joint-to-joint alignment, **move** the image to the side of the screen and use it as a straight edge. Fill out the entire chart NOW before moving on.

Side View Structural Evaluation Chart To Determine Subject's Bad Back Type			
Read each observation carefully, then checkmark the outcome in the row below if it applies. Some columns intentionally list the same "presentation." It is possible to have TWO checkmarks in the same row.			
	Column 1	**Column 2**	**Column 3**
	Observe how subject's EAR lines up with their SHOULDER joint (use mid-joint)		
Row A	____*Check here if ear is **IN FRONT** of shoulder*	____*Check here if ear is **IN FRONT** of shoulder*	____Check here if ear is **EVEN** with shoulder
	Observe how subject's SHOULDER lines up with their HIP joint (use mid-joint)		
Row B	____*Check here if shoulder is **EVEN** with hip*	____*Check here if shoulder is **BEHIND** hip*	____*Check here if shoulder is **IN FRONT** of hip*
	Observe how subject's HIP lines up with their KNEE joint (use mid-joint)		
Row C	____*Check here if hip is **IN FRONT** of knee*	____*Check here if hip is **IN FRONT** of knee*	____*Check here if hip is **EVEN** with knee*
	Observe how subject's KNEE lines up with their ANKLE joint (use mid-joint)		
Row D	____*Check here if knee is **IN FRONT** of ankle*	____*Check here if knee is **EVEN** with ankle*	____*Check here if knee is **EVEN** with ankle*
	Observe the shape of the subject's BUTTOCKS		
Row E	____*Check here if butt is **ROUND** or **FLAT***	____*Check here if butt is **FLAT***	____*Check here if butt is **ROUND***
	Observe subject's HAND to THIGH placement		
Row F	____*Check here if the hand falls **IN FRONT** of thigh or closer to the front than midpoint*	____*Check here if the hand falls **ALONG THE SIDE** of thigh or closer to the midpoint than front*	____*Check here if the hand falls **IN FRONT** of thigh or closer to the front than midpoint*
Row G	**Column 1 Total Checkmark Count____**	**Column 2 Total Checkmark Count____**	**Column 3 Total Checkmark Count____**

At this point, the side view chart should be filled out completely, with each row having 1 or 2 checkmarks. This is vitally important so please confirm this. Next, ensure there is only **ONE** checkmark in row B. That checkmark determines the subject's **correct** Bad Back Type. If row B, column 2 has a checkmark, you are *Boobs Meet Belly.* If row B, column 3 has a checkmark, you are *The Stoop.* If row B, column 1 has a checkmark, you are *Front Loader,* and the variable below applies to you.

Front Loader Variable

If row B determined you were a *Front Loader,* this is your **correct** Bad Back Type. However, you should know that you will **transition** into *Boobs Meet Belly* or *The Stoop.* You can determine which one by the highest count in row G. If column 2 has a higher count than column 3, you will transition into *Boobs Meet Belly.* If column 3 has a higher count than column 2, you will transition into *The Stoop.* If your count is tied, your skeletal structure could go either way. This is your future Bad Back Type if you allow your skeletal structure to degrade. I hope you get motivated to reverse your *Front Loader Type* BEFORE it transitions.

PART II: Determine The Subject's *Quirky's*

To begin, use the subject's front-view picture and the Front View Evaluation Chart (to print the chart, go to our website). Follow the observation instructions given on the chart. For additional guidance, refer to the *Quirky's* detailed in Step 4 and *The Good Back Type* pictures. **See page 10, images 1B, 1D**. This part will be easier to complete if you expand the subject's picture on the phone or tablet. Fill out the entire chart NOW before moving on.

Front View Structural Evaluation Chart To Determine Subject's *Quirky's*

Read each observation carefully, then checkmark the outcome in the row below if it applies. Remember to use the subject's Right or Left, not yours.

Observe subject's head (H) has shifted horizontally Right or Left (like an Egyptian). Check that head and chin are level but off to the side and do not line up with the epi-sternal notch.

H	____Check here if head/chin are shifted sideways to subject's Right	____Check here if head/chin are shifted sideways to subject's Left
Q	Subject has a Right *Quirky Sideways Head*	Subject has a Left *Quirky Sideways Head*

Observe subject's head (H) has rotated Right or Left. Check that head and chin do not line up with the epi-sternal notch, ear may appear more visible, and the chin points toward one shoulder.

H	____Check here if the chin is rotated to subject's Right (see more Left ear)	____Check here if the chin is rotated to subject's Left (see more Right ear)
Q	Subject has a Right *Quirky Twisted Head*	Subject has a Left *Quirky Twisted Head*

Observe subject's head (H) has bent Right or Left. The head may appear diagonally aligned.

H	____Check here if the head is tilted to subject's Right (chin points to Left shoulder)	____Check here if the head is tilted to subject's Left (chin points to Right shoulder)
Q	Subject has a Right *Quirky Tilted Head*	Subject has a Left *Quirky Tilted Head*

Observe subject's shoulders (S) are horizontally level. One may appear HIGHER than the other—that's the *Quirky* **(Q)** shoulder.

S	____Check here if subject's Right Shoulder is higher than the other	____Check here if subject's Left Shoulder is higher than the other
Q	Subject has a Right *Quirky Shoulder*	Subject has a Left *Quirky Shoulder*

Observe subject's pelvis (P) is centered. Compare sides. One hip and forearm will have a smaller gap or no gap—that's the *Quirky* **(Q)** pelvis.

P	____Check here if subject's Right hip is closer to Right forearm	____Check here if subject's Left hip is closer to Left forearm
Q	Subject has a Right *Quirky Pelvis*	Subject has a Left *Quirky Pelvis*

At this point, the front view chart should be filled out completely, with checkmarks placed in rows H, S, or P. Directly below that checkmark listed in row Q is the subject's *Quirky*. The subject may have **more than one** *Quirky* head but **only one** *Quirky* shoulder or pelvis. Remember, if you didn't observe any *Quirky's*, don't panic; the subject may not have any.

Congratulations

Discovering your Bad Back Type and *Quirky's* IS—A—BIG—DEAL! Are you ready to reverse those "signs" and shoot for *The Good Back Type*? Step 7 will lay it all out, and Step 8 will make it a piece of cake!

PS: If you would like your Bad Back Type and *Quirky's* confirmed, visit our website for details (Practitioner Confirmed Structural Evaluation).

Part III

TAKE YOUR BAD BACK AND MAKE IT A GOOD BACK

STEP 7: MASTER THE METHODS TO RESTORE YOUR GOOD BACK

The Big Question

After Kristen, our *Front Loader* volunteer **(See page 54, image 5A)**, returned to her seat, the audience was anxious to learn more about the Bad Back Types. I brought Johnny Bones back to the center of the room, and the crowd went silent. People become "awestruck" when they see Johnny, and with this audience's full attention, I could finish his story (See Step 2).

I began: *Remember, Johnny's obituary informed us that he suffered from whiplash complications for twenty-five years, then died on the surgery table...* I paused... *but how do you suppose a **simple case** of whiplash could be so devastating?* I paused again.

*If you've heard of Whiplash-Associated Disorders (WADs), you might be a lawyer, a healthcare practitioner, or a victim of the condition. Otherwise, you probably wouldn't know that whiplash can cause more than neck pain and headaches. With the sudden jolt of an accident, the head and neck are thrown into **flexion*** (I tucked my chin to my chest), *then **hyperextension*** (I extended my head backward until it rested on my shoulders). *Although whiplash occurs **much faster** than I can demonstrate, that's how neck bones shift, discs bulge or crack, and the Master Curve can straighten, or worse, its alignment can reverse. I showed them an example of a reversed neck curve.* **See page 24, image 2H**.

Folks, that's how a simple bumper-to-bumper accident created never-ending problems for Johnny and eventually sent him to his grave. So here's the BIG QUESTION... If Johnny had restored his neck curve after his accident, could that have changed his fatal outcome? With all eyes fixated on Johnny as I pulled him from his flopped-over rag-doll appearance to an upright position, I answered my own question.

Yes, slowly and steadily, Johnny's Stoop could have been reversed so his ear, shoulder, hip, knee, and ankle joints lined up. Then, toting The Good Back Type, his chronic neck and shoulder pain would have subsided, the agonizing burning sensations radiating down his arms would have disappeared, and he'd be tall, blond, and handsome once again (I surmised the handsome part). *All of that could have been made possible* ***just*** *by restoring his Master Curve* (the MORE important curve to restore).

The Only Way You're Gonna Fix Your *Bowling Ball Head*

Sarah, my assistant, saw that it was demonstration time. From the corner of my eye, I could see she was making her way to the stage with a chair in her hands. She placed the chair sideways, sat down, and waited for my signal. The audience was busily engaged in break-out groups strung across the room and couldn't be bothered to notice.

May I have your attention? Assuming you and your partner have had enough time to evaluate each other for Bowling Ball Head, with a show of hands, who's got that "sign?" Every person raised their hand.

Nice. You ALL have Bowling Ball Head. It's the most common and easiest "sign" to detect of all Bad Back Signs, and if you'll bring your attention to Sarah, she's got the solution to reversing that problem sign.

I gave Sarah the go-ahead nod, and she quickly slid her butt to the middle of her seat, leaned her upper body backward, and lowered her head over the edge of the chair until it was completely hanging freely. The audience watched intently as she wrapped her arms around the back of the chair and clasped her fingers together. Sarah's body sat motionless, her Adam's apple pointed up toward the ceiling, and that's when I said, *This is the ONLY way you're gonna fix your Bowling Ball Head.*

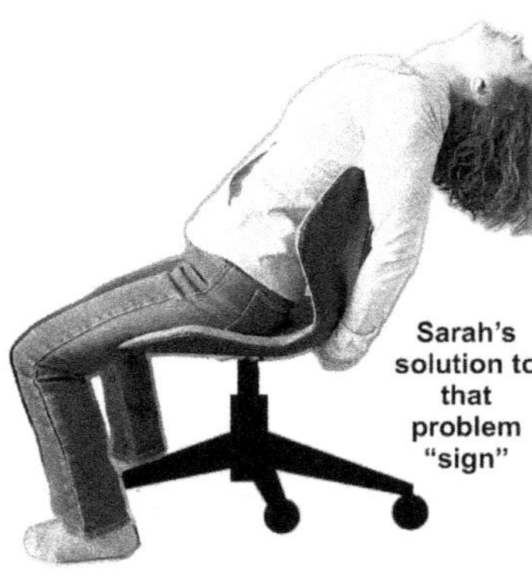

Three Most FAQS

Since all Bad Back Types include *Bowling Ball Head*, it was the ONLY "sign" we taught our audiences how to reverse. It began with Sarah's demonstration, a dramatic but successful attention grabber. With every eye in the room focused on her silent figure draped over the back of the chair, I began instruction by addressing the three most frequently asked questions (FAQS): *What's It Called, What's It Doing, and Why Does It Look So Scary?*

What's It Called

Now that you've discovered your Bad Back Type and maybe a *Quirky* or two, your goal is to make your Bad Back parts, good. The task of going from bad to good will require some restoration work. You will restore the curves to the curvy parts and restore the straight to its bent parts. This process is called The Reverse Strategy Method.

What's It Doing

The Reverse Strategies restore faulty skeletal and backbone parts to their natural alignment by pushing or pulling them into a **stretch**, which **trains** them to **stay in place.** All Bad Back Signs and *Quirky's* can be reversed using a strategy or two, sometimes three. For example, *Bowling Ball Head* requires two parts.

Part I pulls the head and neck bones backward into a stretch to train them to stay on top of the shoulders (Sarah's demonstration). Part II uses an orthopedic device to push the neck bones into a curvy stretch to train them to stay in place.

Why Does It Look So Scary

Do you remember how a Good Back becomes bad? A force moves skeletal and backbone parts out of alignment, and the only way misaligned parts will move back is with another force. Reverse Strategies are that force—a gentle force. Each is designed to push or pull a faulty part into its **natural curvy** or **straight alignment**.

Sarah's demonstration with her head pulled backward might have looked scary and uncomfortable, but she held that stretch for 10 minutes, so rest assured, she wasn't suffering.

REVERSE STRATEGIES FOR ALL BAD BACK TYPES AND *QUIRKY'S*

This is the section you've been patiently waiting for. It's the "how to" reverse your Bad Back Type and *Quirky's*. Follow the strategy list below for YOUR "type." Reverse Strategies for *Quirky's* are listed at the end of this step. The recommendation is to **SKIM** through your strategies and quickly proceed to Step 8, which is packed with ALL the details, explanations, and device information to help you successfully implement your Reverse Strategies.

Front Loader **(FL) Strategy List** (follow only the numbers listed)

- Reverse *Bowling Ball Head* Strategy (#1)
- Reverse *Cold Shoulders* Strategy (#2)
- Reverse *Pelvic Thrust 'n' Tilt* Strategy (#4)

Boobs Meet Belly **(BMB) Strategy List** (follow only the numbers listed)

- Reverse *Bowling Ball Head* Strategy (#1)
- Reverse *HunchBack Shoulders* Strategy (#3)
- Reverse *Pelvic Thrust 'n' Tilt* Strategy (#4)

The Stoop **(ST) Strategy List** (follow only the numbers listed)

- Reverse *Bowling Ball Head* Strategy (#1)
- Reverse *Cold Shoulders* Strategy (#2)
- Reverse *Pelvic Back-Ender w/ Dip* Strategy (#5)

(#1) REVERSE *BOWLING BALL HEAD* STRATEGY (2 PARTS)

PART I: Pull Head Backward (aka *Gravity Monster Solution*): This strategy pulls the head and neck bones backward.

- **Pulling Force:** Gravity.
- **Placement of Body:** Position the body face up, widthwise on a bed, lengthwise on a long ottoman, or a step aerobic bench. The shoulder blades should be supported enough to allow the head and neck to hang freely. For more support, use the shortest Wedge piece under the shoulders.
- **Hold the Molding Stretch:** 1-20 minutes to train the head and neck bones to stay in place and promote the 4 Curve Alignment.

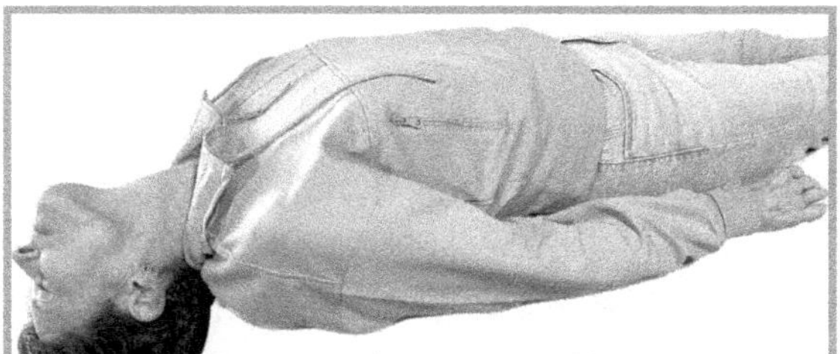

Reverse *Bowling Ball Head* Strategy
Pull Head Backward

PART II: Push Neck Forward: This strategy pushes neck bones forward into the Master Curve (the MORE important curve to restore).

- **Pushing Force Device:** Use any size Newdle, Twodle, or the Tower.
- **Placement of Device and Body:** Place the device horizontally on a bed or the floor (for more resistance). Lay the body face up with the neck on the device. Position the device directly UNDER neck bones #3, #4, and #5 (midpoint of the neck curve). Do not let the skull or shoulders rest on the device. Arms and legs extend.
- **Hold the Molding Stretch:** 1-20 minutes to train the neck bones to stay in place and promote the 4 Curve Alignment.

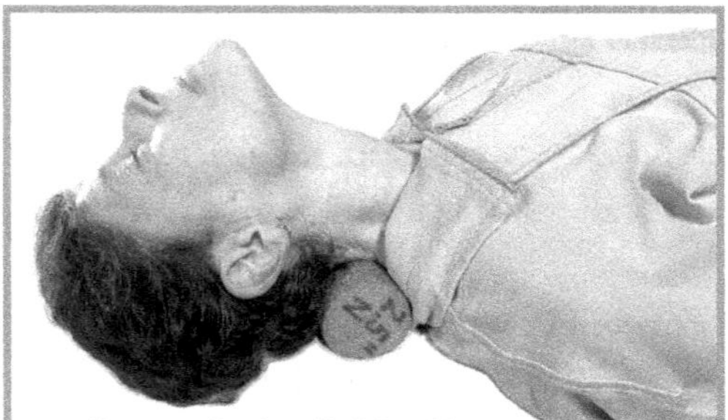

Reverse *Bowling Ball Head* Strategy
Push Neck Forward

(#2) REVERSE *COLD SHOULDERS* STRATEGY (2 PARTS)

PART I: Push Them Backward: This strategy pushes the middle-back and shoulder girdle backward.

- **Pushing Force Device:** Use the Wedged Block. Stack pieces as high as can be tolerated. The Half or Full Moon device is another option.
- **Placement of Device and Body:** Place the device on a bed or the floor (for more resistance). Lay your body face down, with the upper body directly on the device (high side) so that the ribcage rests on the device just UNDER the chest (breasts hang over the edge of the Wedge or Moon, upper body angles upward). Legs are extended, elbows resting on the floor while hands lay flat or support the chin.
- **Hold the Molding Stretch:** 1-20 minutes to train the middle-back bones and shoulder girdle to stay in place and promote the 4 Curve Alignment.

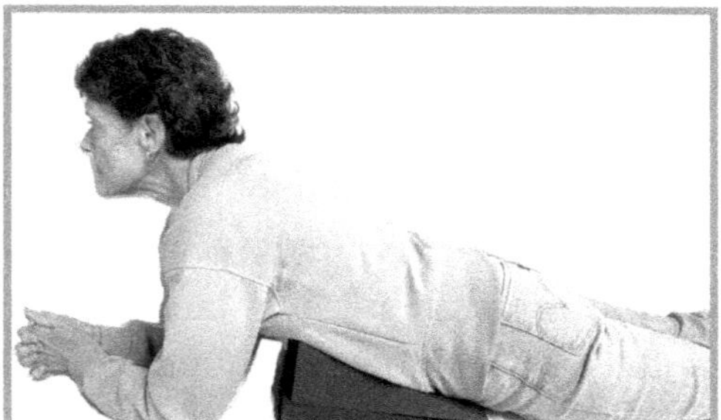

Reverse *Cold Shoulders* Strategy
Push Them Backward

PART II: Push Middle-Back Forward: This strategy pushes the middle-back forward. Optional but recommended for BMB "types."

- **Pushing Force Device:** Use the SHORTEST length Newdle or Twodle. This device is easiest to "place" by inserting it inside your clothing to secure it before molding the middle-back.
- **Placement of Device and Body:** Place the device vertically, BETWEEN the shoulder blades (not touching neck bones). Lay the body face up with the middle-back directly on the device, on a bed, or the floor (for more resistance). Arms and legs extended.
- **Hold the Molding Stretch:** 1-20 minutes to train the middle-back bones to stay in place and promote the 4 Curve Alignment.

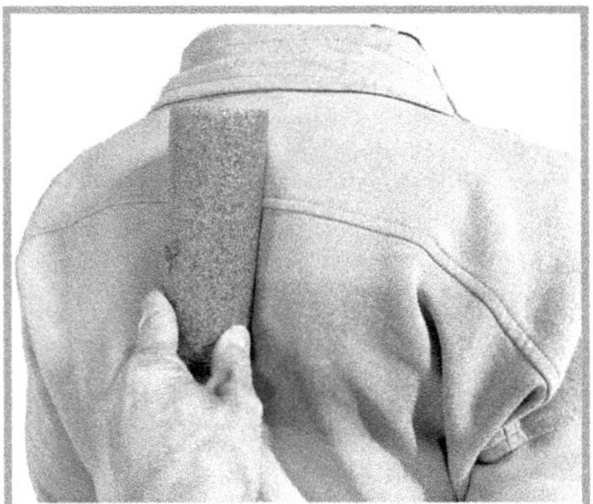

Reverse *Cold Shoulders* Strategy
Push Middle-Back Forward

(#3) REVERSE *HUNCHBACK SHOULDERS* STRATEGY (1 PART)

PART I: Push Them Forward: This strategy pushes the middle-back and shoulder girdle forward.

- **Pushing Force Device:** Use the Wedged Block. Stack pieces as high as can be tolerated. The Half or Full Moon device is another option.
- **Placement of Device and Body:** Place the device on the EDGE of a bed, long ottoman, or step aerobic bench. Lay the body face up with the middle-back directly on the device so that the shoulder blades are placed ACROSS (high side). Shoulder blades

should be supported enough to allow the head and neck to hang freely. If this is not possible, let the head rest on the bed or floor.

- **Hold the Molding Stretch:** 1-20 minutes to train the middle-back bones and shoulder girdle to stay in place and promote the 4 Curve Alignment.

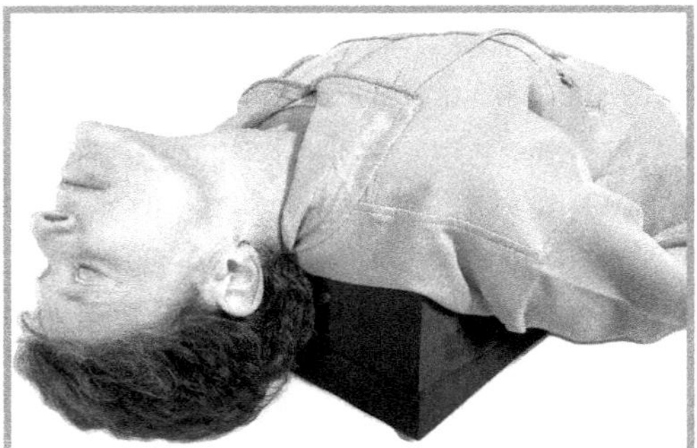

Reverse *HunchBack Shoulders* Strategy
Push Them Forward

(#4) REVERSE *PELVIC THRUST 'N' TILT* STRATEGY (3 PARTS)

PART I: Push Pelvis Backward: This strategy pushes the pelvic girdle backward.

- **Pushing Force:** Use the Wedged Block. Stack pieces as high as can be tolerated. The Half or Full Moon device is another option.
- **Placement of Device and Body:** Place the device on a bed or the floor (for more resistance). Lay face down with the lower body directly on the device so that the pelvis rests ACROSS the device (high side) just BELOW the belly (hangs over the edge of the Wedge or Moon, butt in the air). Legs extended, rest the chin on a pillow, and DON'T rotate the head.
- **Hold the Molding Stretch:** 1-20 minutes to train the pelvis to stay in place and promote the 4 Curve Alignment.

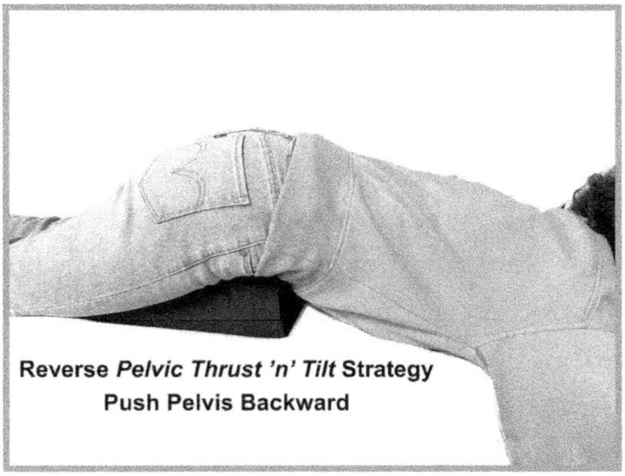

Reverse *Pelvic Thrust 'n' Tilt* Strategy
Push Pelvis Backward

PART II: Push Sacrum Forward: This strategy pushes the sacrum to DIP forward.

- **Pushing Force Device:** Use the SHORTEST length Newdle or Twodle. This device is easiest to "place" by inserting it inside your clothing to secure it before molding the sacrum.
- **Placement of Device and Body:** Place the device vertically BETWEEN the butt cheeks (not touching low-back bones or coccyx). Lay the body face up with the pelvis directly on the device on a bed or the floor (for more resistance). Arms and legs extended.
- **Hold the Molding Stretch:** 1-20 minutes to train the sacrum to stay in place and promote the 4 Curve Alignment.

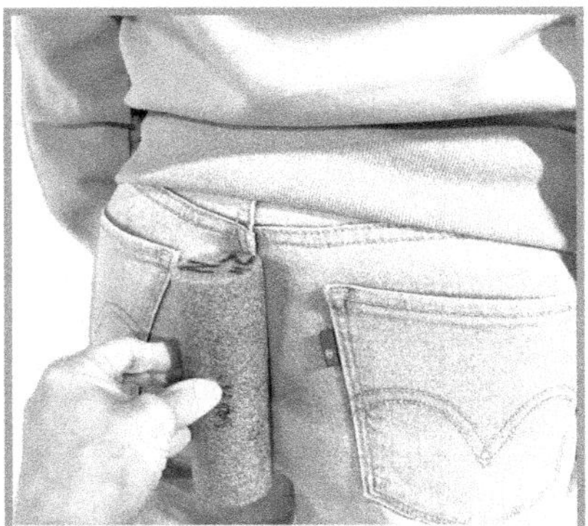

Reverse *Pelvic Thrust 'n' Tilt* Strategy
Push Sacrum Forward

PART III: Push Low-Back Forward: This strategy pushes the low-back into the Master Curve (the MORE important curve to restore).

- **Pushing Force Device:** Use any size Newdle or Twodle.
- **Placement of Device and Body:** Place the device horizontally on a bed or the floor (for more resistance). Lay the body face up with the low-back directly on the device. Position the device UNDER the low-back bones #2, #3, and #4 (midpoint of the curve). Do not let the sacral base rest on the device. Arms and legs extended.
- **Hold the Molding Stretch:** 1-20 minutes to train the low-back bones to stay in place and promote the 4 Curve Alignment.

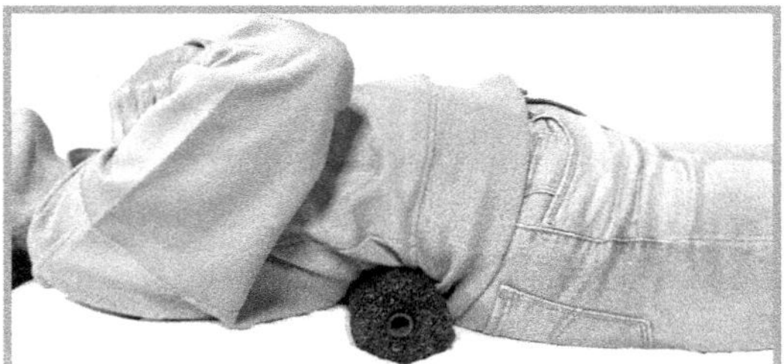

Reverse *Pelvic Thrust 'n' Tilt* Strategy
Reverse *Pelvic Back-Ender w/ Dip* Strategy
Push Low-Back Forward
(Image 7A)

(#5) REVERSE *PELVIC BACK-ENDER W/ DIP* STRATEGY (2 PARTS)

PART I: Push Pelvis Forward: This strategy pushes the pelvic girdle forward and pushes the sacrum to TILT backward.

- **Pushing Force:** Use the Wedged Blocks. Stack pieces as high as can be tolerated. The Half or Full Moon device is another option.
- **Placement of Device and Body:** Place the device on a bed or the floor (for more resistance). Lay the body face up with the lower-body directly on the device so that the butt cheeks rest ACROSS the device (high side). Arms and legs extend downward.
- **Hold the Molding Stretch:** 1-20 minutes to train the pelvis and sacrum to stay in place and promote the 4 Curve Alignment.

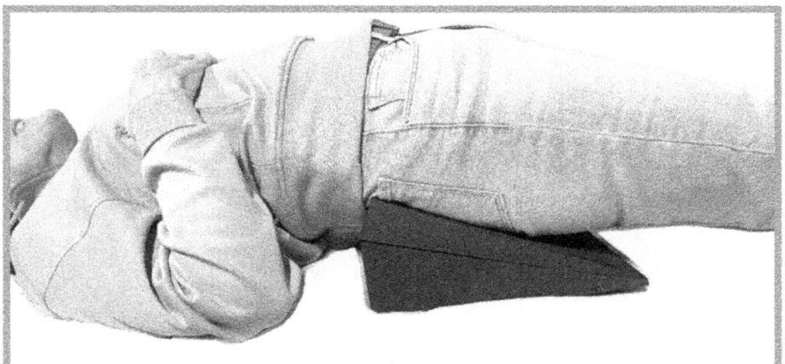

Reverse *Pelvic Back-Ender w/ Dip* Strategy
Push Pelvis Forward

PART II: Push Low-Back Forward: This strategy pushes the low-back into the Master Curve (the MORE important curve to restore). **See page 92, image 7A.**

- **Pushing Force Device:** Use any size Newdle or Twodle.
- **Placement of Device and Body:** Place the device horizontally on a bed or the floor (for more resistance). Lay the body face up with the low-back directly on the device. Position the device UNDER the low-back bones #2, #3, and #4 (midpoint of the curve). Do not let the sacral base rest on the device. Arms and legs extended.
- **Hold the Molding Stretch:** 1-20 minutes to train the low-back bones to stay in place and promote the 4 Curve Alignment.

REVERSE *QUIRKY SIDE-WAYS HEAD* STRATEGY

PART I: Push Head Opposite: This strategy pushes the *Quirky Head* to the opposite side.

- **Pushing Force:** Use the Wedged Blocks or Moons.
- **Placement of Device and Body:** Place the device horizontally on a bed or the floor (for more resistance). Lay the body sideways with the *Quirky Head* (shifted side) on the device, not the neck.
- **Hold the Molding Stretch:** 5-20 minutes to train the head and neck bones to stay in place and promote their centered and Vertically Straight Alignment.

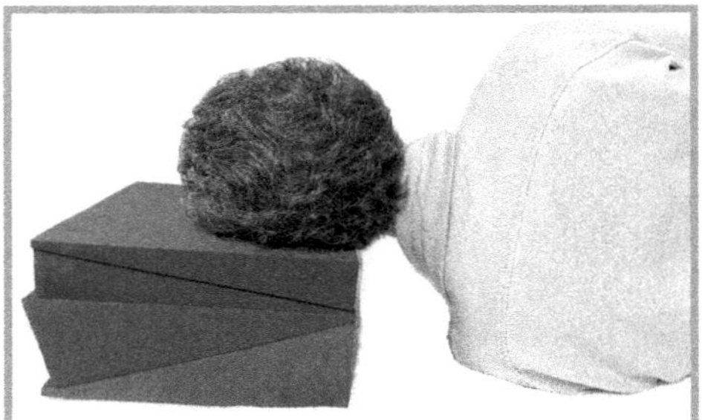

Reverse *Quirky Sideways Head* Strategy
Push Head Opposite

REVERSE *QUIRKY TWISTED HEAD* STRATEGY

PART I: Twist Head Opposite: This strategy twists the *Quirky Head* in the opposite direction.

- **Pushing Force:** Muscle tension.
- **Placement of Body:** Standing is easiest (arms extended downward). Rotate the *Quirky Head* (twisted side) to the opposite side (keep shoulders level); tense (squeeze) neck muscles.
- **Hold the Molding Stretch:** Hold muscle tension for 5 slow-deep breaths in and out of the nose, 3-5x per day. (Step 8, Rule #6, Mold in the Bathroom). This strategy trains the head and neck bones to stay in place and promote their centered and Vertically Straight Alignment.

REVERSE *QUIRKY TILTED HEAD* STRATEGY

PART I: Tilt Head Opposite: This strategy tilts the *Quirky Head* in the opposite direction.

- **Pushing Force:** Muscle tension.
- **Placement of Body:** Standing is easiest (arms extended downward). Bend the *Quirky Head* (tilted side) to the opposite side (keep shoulders level); tense (squeeze) neck muscles.

- **Hold the Molding Stretch:** Hold muscle tension for 5 slow-deep breaths in and out of the nose, 3-5x per day. (Step 8, Rule #6, Mold in the Bathroom). This strategy trains the head and neck bones to stay in place and promote their centered and Vertically Straight Alignment.

REVERSE *QUIRKY SHOULDER* STRATEGY

PART I: Pull Shoulder Down: This strategy pulls the *Quirky Shoulder* downward.

- **Pulling Force:** Muscle tension.
- **Placement of Body:** Standing is easiest (arms extended downward). Pull ONLY the *Quirky Shoulder* (high side) downward (do not bend the head or upper body); tense (squeeze) the shoulder muscles.
- **Hold the Molding Stretch:** Hold muscle tension for 5 slow-deep breaths in and out of the nose, 3-5x per day. (Step 8, Rule #6, Mold in the Bathroom). This strategy trains the *Quirky Shoulder* to stay in place and promote middle-back Vertically Straight Alignment.

REVERSE *QUIRKY PELVIC* STRATEGY

PART I: Push Pelvis Opposite: This strategy pushes the *Quirky Pelvis* to the opposite side.

- **Pushing Force:** Use the Wedged Block. Stack as high as can be tolerated. The Half or Full Moon device is another option.
- **Placement of Device and Body:** Place the device horizontally on a bed or the floor (for more resistance). Lay the body sideways with the *Quirky Pelvis* (shifted side) on the device (use high-side). Place a pillow under the head so it's in a neutral position, and bend the knees.

- **Hold the Molding Stretch:** 5-20 minutes to train the *Quirky Pelvis* to stay in place and promote its centered alignment and low-back and sacrum Vertically Straight Alignment.

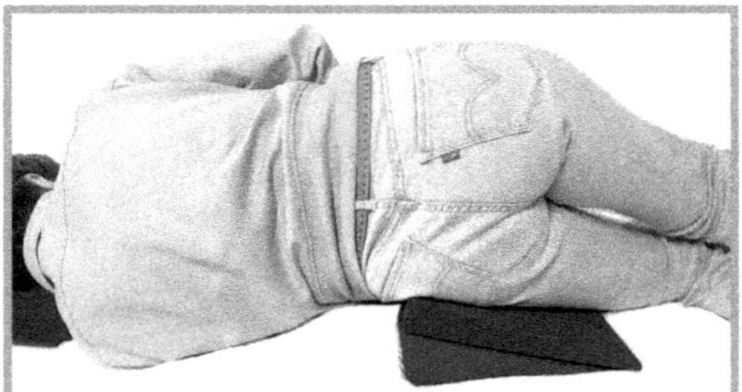

Reverse *Quirky Pelvis* Strategy
Push Pelvis Opposite

My Mother—Years Later

I had almost finished writing this book when, out of the blue, my mother sent me a text with an X-ray of her backbone, including her pelvis and replaced hip—how timely! Unfortunately, Mom had a motor vehicle accident just days prior, which was why she had the image taken. It's been **eight years** since Mom fell from her porch chair, which resulted in a Right hip fracture. See page 49, An Active Woman.

(Image 7B)

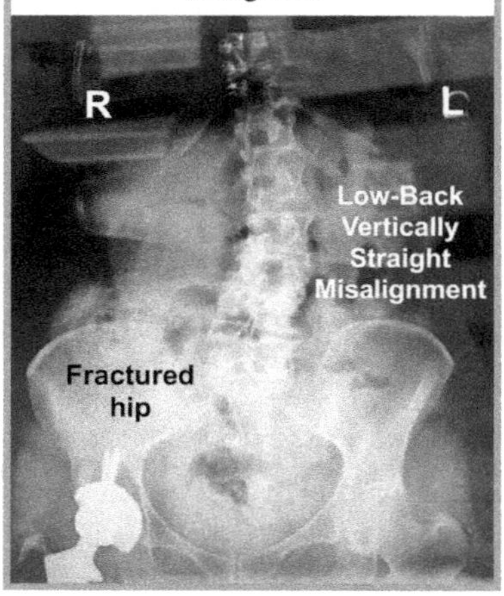

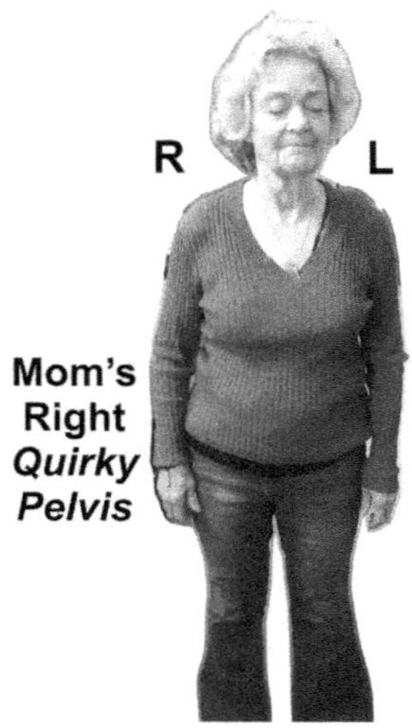

You should be able to detect Mom's hip replacement and her low-back Vertically Straight Misalignment. That misalignment looks like scoliosis, and because we can see degeneration and bone spurs, we know it's been there a long time. Nevertheless, Mom's case makes a good lesson. *See how her pelvis shifted to the Right to create that smidgen of light between her Left forearm and hip?* Mom's Right *Quirky Pelvis* is not centered and has always caused Mom to be off balance (she walks into walls, bumps her hip on the corner of the kitchen table, and sits cock-eyed in chairs).

It's too bad Mom didn't use the device I had recommended. If she had placed it under her *Quirky Pelvis,* she might have trained her pelvic girdle to stay center-aligned. Since the pelvis is a significant part of the body, helping it to stay in its natural alignment could have restored her balance, and she might have walked and sat a little straighter.

Restore Balance

When the ear, shoulder, hip, knee, and ankle joints line up in *The Good Back Type*, the skeletal structure is BALANCED (aka stable). But because you've got *Front Loader*, *Boobs Meet Belly*, or *The Stoop Bad Back Type* you've got 3 faulty skeletal parts (head, shoulders, pelvis) and 4 faulty backbone parts (neck, middle-back, low-back, sacrum), plus *Quirky's*, throwing you OUT OF BALANCE (aka unstable).

The whole idea behind using an orthopedic device (as recommended by each Reverse Strategy) is to push those faulty parts back into their natural alignment to *restore balance* (stability). This is the ONLY goal of *The Bad Back To Good Back Method.* When the misaligned parts are **trained** to stay in their *correct alignment*, joints can **function,** but left in an *incorrect alignment,* joints can **malfunction**, and eventually, they degenerate.

Sadly, that was the story with Mom's hip. My 83-year-old health-nut-hippie of a Mother is STILL very active. She walks her dog, eats homemade foods, and takes lots of vitamins... unfortunately... all that good stuff couldn't save her hip joint. Maybe the Wedged Blocks I gave her the year before her accident could have helped.

DEGENERATIVE JOINT DISEASE (DJD) is a condition that can affect any skeletal joint but strikes weight-bearing joints more often (hips, knees, feet). When the pelvis is forced to shift from its centered alignment, the "load" becomes unequally distributed. Some joints aren't stressed, while others have to "bear more load," and those joints are more likely to **jam**…

MAKE A—> Fist with both hands and ram them together, that's a **jammed** joint. If you don't release that stress, your fists will turn white and eventually go numb because the joints can't get proper nerve energy. It's the same with any of your jammed joints. If the pressure remains, nerve energy decreases, inflammation sets in, gets trapped, and attracts bacteria and viruses. That's when things go south. Joint fluid thickens like rubber cement, and movement becomes more difficult, but somehow, you continue to use and even overuse the rubbing, grinding, painful, and **stuck** joints. Exercise and medications usually override discomfort or dysfunction, but joints continue to degenerate. The situation might improve if the pelvic girdle is trained to stay center-aligned.

HIP FRACTURE is a break in the femur head (or femoral neck) most likely caused by degeneration. When these 2 pelvic joints have to BEAR more load over a long period of time, they become vulnerable to injury.

LIKE WITH—> My mother's case, long before her traumatic fall, she was *The Stoop.* Coupled with her *Quirky Pelvis,* Mom's weight-bearing joints were stressed for a long time. *Wonder why I wasn't able to help her?* Interestingly enough, Mom didn't have ANY back, hip, or leg pain. Without pain, she wasn't motivated to do anything about her Bad Back, not even the easy molding stretches I gave her the year before her accident. Unfortunately, surgery isn't designed to correct Bad Back Types or *Quirky's,* so Mom STILL has *The Stoop* and a *Quirky Pelvis,* only now, **they** are worse.

SCOLIOSIS is a condition resulting from multiple Vertically Straight Misalignments.

I'VE HELPED—> Many *scoliosis* patients in my career, so I know firsthand that correcting a single or double curvature takes lots of time and effort for both practitioner and patient. Still, there's no guarantee bones will stack solidly and squarely one on top of the other. Instead of oodles of office visits and bracing devices, we Bad Back "typed" our *scoliosis* patients, identified their *Quirky's*, and set them on a course to make their Bad Back good. That was our protocol, and it helped return the strength, stability, and springy-ness to their scoliotic structure.

After reviewing your Reverse Strategies, you should be excited but may be slightly overwhelmed. Don't worry… taking your Bad Back and making it a Good Back is well worth the effort! The 13 Rules you are about to learn are designed to make reversing your Bad Back Type and *Quirky's* easy—so—get ready—get set—GO!

STEP 8: FOLLOW THE GOOD BACK RULES

RULE #1—YOUR STRATEGIES ARE YOURS FOR LIFE

This rule states that the strategies designed to reverse your Bad Back Type are yours, and they're yours for life. Let me clarify. Your Bad Back Type isn't here today and gone in a month or two just because you lay your head over a device every day. Your skeletal structure shifted over many years, and to shift it back will take many years. *How many years?*

Taking your Bad Back and making it a Good Back can happen when you use the Reverse Strategies and mold for **twelve months straight**. At that time, you should be able to stand in *The Good Back Type* naturally (without forcing yourself) and join *The Good Back Club*. To continue enjoying your strong, stable, and springy skeletal structure, you must ensure it doesn't shift back into its old *pattern*, and that means you must let it CURE (the process of maintaining placement), which will likely take **another twelve months**.

Realistically, expect the restoration process to take **two years**, but *here's the snag:* gravity's force continually pulls your skeletal structure downward. To cancel out gravity's tug and keep your Good Back good, you should continue to mold for as long as you want to remain upright, tall, straight, and proud with your head held high. This rule recommends making your Reverse Strategies part of your LIFE for... the... rest... of... your... LIFE!

The Fountain of Youth

For our new patients, we taught the Reverse Strategies in a group-style class. A mother and her sixteen-year-old daughter, Claudia, were in attendance. Claudia was plagued with headaches that she blamed on her *Bowling Ball Head* and playing the flute for most of her youth.

Excitedly, she told the class that she hadn't had a single headache since she began hanging her head nightly off her Wedge, then confessed, *"It's so comfortable, I fall asleep!"* At the very next moment, one of our elder patients, Florence, who liked to join our class from time to time, unprompted, stood from her seat in the audience to share her testimony.

> *"I've been coming here for three years, every March through November because I don't drive in the winter. It took me a year to get comfortable hanging my head freely off the Wedge, but now I can do* ***all*** *twenty minutes! In the beginning, I could only mold about thirty seconds. Then I realized I could do thirty seconds, three, four, and five times a day. I just wish someone had told me about this method when I was younger because I'm almost eighty, and I'm molding through severe arthritis. But I can walk through the grocery store without holding onto a cart, my knees don't hurt like they used to, and my children tell me I no longer look like an old lady. This method works, and the best part is that you don't need anybody's help to do it; you only need the courage to get started and commitment to stick with it. If I can do this, anybody can!"*

The class broke out in applause. I thanked Flo, then said:

> *"Speaking of youth, did any of you know these strategies are the fountain of youth? Take Bowling Ball Head, for instance: the more forward the head shifts, the more the throat skin stretches and sags. If you want to make your chin skin disappear, train your head to sit back up and over your shoulders. No products, pills, or potions can promise to keep you upright, resist the pulling effects of gravity, or help you keep the spring in your step more than staying committed to your strategies for life. Congratulations, you've discovered the fountain of youth."*

RULE #2—FITTING YOU WITH A PUSHING FORCE

As discussed, the Reverse Strategies are designed to shift faulty parts toward their natural alignment. To accomplish this task will require a *pushing force*, and this rule introduces you to the orthopedic devices that will *do the pushing*. The devices listed below have been thoroughly tested and successfully used by thousands of patients. During my practicing days, I was the one who helped fit patients with their devices. Now, it's your job to FIT YOURSELF with a suitably sized device as you begin molding and throughout the molding process.

Getting off to a good start with just the right device is vitally important, as that will increase your probability of success. Nothing is worse than using a device sized too big, which would make molding vastly uncomfortable and too difficult to continue. A device sized too small would make molding comfortable and pleasantly easy, which isn't a bad thing**... however...** you could be wasting your time because intensity is necessary to get ligaments and bones to move (Rule #7, Steadily Increase The Push). The challenge to **fitting you** with "just the right device" is that there ISN'T one size that fits all or one device that does it all. *Where do you start?* First, familiarize yourself with the recommended devices below, then go to our website for additional details.

NEWDLE (say new-dull) **DEVICES**

Newdles got their name because molding is new to you, and they look like pool noodles. Use these devices to start the molding process. Each Newdle is a solid, cylinder-shaped tube made of a porous material that squishes slightly when laid upon. This set offers 3 sizes: **2-inch, 2 1/2 inch, 2 3/4 inch**. These sizes support all 4 curves, and children can benefit from them.

TWODLE (say two-dull) **DEVICES**

Twodles are for those ready to UP-SIZE from the Newdle. They are a cylinder-shaped, two-piece device (hence their name) whose core is plugged with a hard tube (for more resistance) and a soft rubber outer layer that squishes when laid upon. This set offers 3 sizes: **2-inch, 2 3/4 inch, 3 1/4 inch**. These sizes support all 4 curves. The **3 1/4 inch** supports the low-back curve only.

WEDGED BLOCK SET

These stiff foam devices support the shoulder and pelvic girdle strategies. Each piece can be used as a single or stacked to offer more height. Use the shorter piece (height) under the shoulders (to create more resistance) for *Gravity Monster Solution*. This set offers 2 sizes: **2-inch, 4-inch**.

TOWER DEVICE

This orthopedic device is designed exclusively for molding the neck and for those ready to UP-SIZE from the **2 3/4 inch** Twodle. The Tower offers additional height and a stiffer material that "increase the push" at the target sight and help to restore the Master Curve.

MOONS

These orthopedic devices are designed for shoulder and pelvic girdle strategies, but NOT for molding the neck or low-back curves. They are wide, solid, cylinder-shaped rolls made of a soft, porous material that squishes slightly. Half moon has one flat side. These devices are best used when molding on the FLOOR. This set offers 2 sizes: **Half Moon 3-inch and Full Moon 6-inch**

A Washcloth or Hand Towel

If you can't tolerate any suggested device, use one or two washcloths or a single hand towel. Fold the cloth in half lengthwise, roll it up as tight as possible, and secure it with rubber bands. Additionally, a folded cloth is the perfect solution under a device to increase its height.

Make Your Own Contraption

Bob was a middle-aged big teddy bear of a guy who drove a delivery truck and blamed his chronic low-back pain on the many hours logged behind the wheel sitting on a squishy seat with metal springs. Bob had *Boobs Meet Belly* and an inconsistent schedule, so his office visits were sporadic. When the holiday season came around, Bob's schedule changed, and we didn't see him for three months straight. One Saturday morning in early March, Bob showed up carrying a triangular wooden contraption. Excitedly, he walked to the front desk and firmly placed it down with a thud, drawing everybody's attention. It was literally a stack of 2x4s screwed together and wrapped in foam.

> *"Dr. Faith, I made this because I was getting too comfortable with the foam device you gave me, and my schedule wouldn't allow me to come in. I lay over this sturdy triangle every night while listening to the Ten O' Clock News, and I haven't had any low-back pain!"*

Then, as if the whole office hadn't already overheard his declaration (we had an open-concept office), he turned to face the room filled with patients.

> *"Good people, I'm here to tell you this stuff works. My doctor told me I'd have to live with my back pain as long as I drove a truck, but he was wrong. Listen to Dr. Faith, she knows her stuff!"*

Bob hugged me, grabbed his contraption, and walked out. We never saw Bob again.

Fitting You With A Suitable Size

Let me point out that you can't make a wrong decision as you attempt to fit your long neck, broad shoulders, or big butt with a device. Keep trying out sizes until you find the right one that "challenges the target site" but doesn't make you feel like giving up! Additionally, don't be afraid to get creative. The devices listed above can be found on our website, and they are highly effective, but if a bundle of 2x4s works for you, *good golly,* use it!

RULE #3—GET TO 5 BUT SHOOT FOR 20

This rule states that the primary objective of each Reverse Strategy is to mold for at least 5 minutes, but make 20 minutes your ultimate GOAL. This may sound easier than it is.

Let me explain: each molding stretch is designed to push or pull a faulty skeletal or backbone part into a stretch. That means that for every part being stretched, the counterpart will have to be shortened. For instance, when you lay your head over the side of the bed for *Gravity Monster Solution*, the ligaments and muscles in the front of your neck are forced to stretch, while the ligaments and muscles in the back of your neck are forced to shorten. To get the ligaments and muscles to conform to the Reverse Strategy, they MUST BE stretched or shortened, which depends solely on *CREEP.*

How To Work *WITH CREEP* And Not Against It

So, I'm not referring to creepy things or the creeps in your life. Creep is a physiological phenomenon of soft tissue (ligaments and muscles) that makes molding for any length of time easy or challenging. With a brief tutorial on muscles, ligaments, and creep, you will better understand

WHY this rule recommends molding for 5 minutes but shooting for 20.

Let's begin: ligaments are strong but flexible connective tissue that connect bone to bone, like the thigh bone to the leg (knee joint) or the arm bone to the forearm (elbow joint). These cartilaginous fibers are mostly a **plastic** material with a small amount of elastic, like your favorite pair of stretchy jeans: 98% cotton and 2% spandex. Ligaments are arranged in short, fibrous strands that interlace for strength and durability. Follow the exercise below to understand *how ligaments creep.*

Try This —> Take both hands, palms facing you, fingertips facing each other. Interlace your fingers sideways until you can't push them together any further (thumbs up). This is how ligaments are arranged, parallel to each other, with their fibers interlaced. Notice that because your fingers are tightly held together, they would be strong against something that tried to plow through them. Now, pull your hands apart s-l-o-w-l-y so your fingers begin to separate, exposing the space between them. That's how ligament fibers **creep** to **stretch**. The further separated your fingers get, the WEAKER the ligaments would be against that same plow, and that's how bone can easily shift OUT of its curvy, straight, or centered alignment. If you were to s-l-o-w-l-y push your fingers back together, that's how ligament fibers **creep** to **shorten**.

Ligament fibers that were forced to **creep/stretch** weakened (so bone has the opportunity to shift), but those same fibers can be forced to **creep/shorten** and become strong again (so bone stays in place). That's how the Reverse Strategies work and it's how YOU are going to restore your faulty parts, but before you do, you MUST understand how—to—work—***WITH—CREEP***—and—not—against—it.

CREEP Starts At Five

It cannot be emphasized enough how ALL Reverse Strategies must be directed toward getting the ligaments to creep/stretch. That is how bones are encouraged to return to their natural alignment. *Are you wondering if muscles have a hand in restoring the bone?* They do, but muscles aren't a plastic material like ligaments. Muscle fibers are mostly **elastic**, like a rubber band, and therefore can be stretched more easily. Here's how an experiment conducted decades ago gave researchers some amazing insight into how muscles and ligaments respond when they are forced to hold a stretch.

Study subjects: hung their head freely off the end of an exam table with a harness strapped under their chin and a three-pound weight attached. For subjects who could handle this *barbaric trial* for 5 minutes, scientists noted their neck **muscles** actively stretched during that time. For subjects who "hung in there" longer, scientists noted their neck **ligaments** began stretching AFTER 5 minutes but stopped stretching AFTER 20 minutes. From this study, researchers concluded that two distinct phases occur during a molding stretch:

- **The Elastic Phase** occurs from 0-5 minutes of a molding stretch. During this 5-minute period, muscle fibers creep/stretch, so muscles will "bark," and discomfort is likely.
- **The Plastic Phase** occurs from 5–20 minutes of a molding stretch. During this 15-minute period, ligament fibers creep/stretch, and muscles settle down, so molding is easier.

The Upshot: if you can hold that molding stretch for ALL 5 minutes and get through the elastic phase despite "barking" muscles, GOOD. If you can easily and comfortably hold that molding stretch for 20 minutes and get through the plastic phase when creep/stretch occurs, and ligaments conform to the mold, EXCELLENT.

Ligaments begin to creep/stretch after 5 minutes and stop creeping at 20 minutes, so **hold that molding stretch** with this goal in mind;

otherwise, you won't restore a curve or restore the straight; you will ONLY be stretching muscles.

My Cousin's Floppy Ears

When I was about eight years old, my family took a trip over the Thanksgiving holiday to see my Aunt Jo and her four kids. When we arrived, we were surprised to see little Brad, who was about two years old, running around excitedly. That's probably not unusual for a toddler, but the masking tape placed over his ears was quite a sight. Quickly, my aunt responded to our stares by whispering. *"Ignore his ears and treat Brad like everything's normal."* She promised to fill us in later.

When "later" arrived, she asked us to recall that Brad's ears flopped outward. She hoped that taping them to his head would re-train them. Now, as I look back on my aunt's training methods, it would seem a logical approach, especially since Bradley wore a baseball cap to hold his taped-up ears in place, but science doesn't support the outcome she was hoping for. You see, ligaments of the ear are not that different from the ones that hold the Backbones together, and to get either of them to do what you want, they MUST be placed under stress. When ligament fibers are stressed, they will *creep*.

Q: *How do you stress ligament fibers?*

A: Push, bend, twist, or flex them in the opposite direction from which they currently exist. That would qualify as *forced stress*. The ligament fibers would stretch or shorten, conform, and eventually stay in place.

In the case of my cousin's ears, which needed to go from floppy to vertical, Aunt Jo should have folded Brad's ears in half (toward his head) and kept them taped up for 20 minutes every day for a year (and another year to cure). That stress would have forced his ear fibers to conform to the desired position; and *disrupt the old way* in an effort to be *arranged in a new way*. As I remember, when we saw my cousins again in the spring, Brad's ears were still floppy, but no tape or baseball hat. My Aunt Jo had given up.

The Moral Of The Story

The same is true for *Bowling Ball Head.* To get the head to sit back on top of the shoulders, it has to be held backward (extension) from its current forward position for 20 minutes every day for a year, and another year to cure. That molding stretch would force the ligament fibers in the front of the neck to creep/stretch and the ligament fibers in the back of the neck to creep/shorten. Eventually, the head and neck bones would **shift** and **stay** in their natural alignment.

RULE #4—HOLD THAT MOLDING STRETCH

This rule recommends holding each Reverse Strategy for 1 minute and increasing in 1-minute increments until you can easily and comfortably hold that molding stretch for all 20 minutes in a single session. You may wonder if starting with a minute and advancing a minute at a time is too cautious. No, it's not; it's realistic.

Whether you reach the 20-minute goal in 20 days or 20 weeks doesn't matter. Some individuals can dive right in, but most must mind their bodies and proceed slowly. The amount of time you can hold that molding stretch will depend on how well your muscles, tendons, ligaments, and bones can handle being pushed and pulled. Use the recommendations below to guide you with a steadily increasing molding pace.

Setting A Timer can help you manage your molding minutes and track a steady increase. Like setting a timer to help you avoid burning cookies baking in the oven, set a timer to help you avoid spending more time molding than your muscles can handle. You **can** overcook yourself during a session, and you'd easily know because the next day, your muscles would literally be on fire! Especially in the beginning, **ease** into molding with the help of a timer and gradually increase your molding minutes.

Listen To Your Body it will tell you how long it's willing to *hold that molding stretch.* Whether you're hanging your head off the bed *(Gravity Monster Solution)* or your low-back is stretched over a Twodle (Push

Low-Back Forward), you will begin to get uncomfortable. That is your body telling you; it's almost quitting time. If you don't end your molding session right then, you will get **really** uncomfortable. That is your body telling you, IT'S HAD ENOUGH. Scootch down your Wedge or roll off your Twodle and **end** your molding session.

END your Molding Session if you feel nauseous, the back of your head goes numb, you experience dizziness, or molding is "downright impossible." These symptoms usually indicate bony pressure on the brain stem, so DON'T try to tough it out. More frequent molding sessions for shorter periods of time should alleviate these episodes. If symptoms persist, getting an Adjustment can help, and this is especially true for the "downright impossible" cases (Step 9, Backbone Therapy).

Take A Molding Break if your muscles get SO achy and sore you just can't continue. Especially in the beginning, your muscles WILL react to being pushed and pulled. If the muscle spasms get SO bad, you'll need to take a molding break until "things" calm down. One or two days is usually sufficient, but don't stress over taking "more time off" if needed. Massage can help (Step 9, Soft Tissue Therapy).

Don't Take A Molding Break that's too long. This advice is probably the most important, whether you are just beginning or have been molding for years. If you let too much time lapse between molding sessions, such as two weeks or more, you increase the likelihood of experiencing muscle soreness, trigger points, and tension headaches when you resume. It's no fun dealing with trigger points and tension headaches over and over again; to avoid that scenario, DON'T STOP MOLDING.

Molding Time Adds Up means the amount of time you mold within 24 hours goes toward your total minute count. For instance, you mold for 3 minutes, 4x in one day; that's 12 minutes. After 24 hours, you'll start back at zero. Mold as often as you can fit into a day until you can *hold that molding stretch* for 20 minutes STRAIGHT. If you can't tolerate a certain molding stretch, you'll have to proceed more slowly. Try molding for any length of time (say 30 seconds), three, four, and five times daily, and keep increasing.

Weak Muscle Myth

Many times during my career, patients would tell me their practitioner, therapist, or trainer told them their back problems were caused by weak stomach or back muscles and advised them to *get to the gym*. In most cases, this actually "did the trick," and back problems seemed to disappear—*or did they?*

One cannot dispute the fact that walking, running (aerobics), lifting weights (strength), and yoga (stretching) can help keep muscles toned, joints flexible, and blood, lymph, and oxygen circulating. Exercising in any form is good, but back problems MUST be blamed on a weak skeletal structure (a Bad Back Type). The "trick" to strengthening the skeletal structure is identifying its weakest parts (aka faulty parts). Then, push, bend, twist, fold, or flex them in the opposite direction from which they currently exist; *hold that stretch* for twenty minutes every day for a year and another year to cure.

This is not a myth: restore the curves, restore the straight, and reap the benefits.

RULE #5—HEAT 'EM UP TO MOLD AND MOVE 'EM

Before your ligaments can begin to budge, you must get the muscles to stretch during the first 5 minutes of molding. You can help that process by using an external heating source to warm up the soft tissue. *Here's the logic:* when muscles and ligaments are warm, their fibers can move more easily. That's why hot yoga is so popular. Yoga students can get a deeper stretch when the studio temperature is 85º. Before you *hold that molding stretch*, try these suggestions:

- Bean Bags filled with beans, flaxseed, or corn can be heated in the microwave and applied for 10-15 minutes before your molding session. I don't recommend electric heating pads because they interfere with the body's natural current.

- A blanket to cover yourself while you mold can help keep the body warm, which naturally cools, as you lay motionless over your device.
- Heat the room with a space heater, mold in front of a fireplace, or in a sauna.

Ligaments Are Like Hockey Sticks

When our middle son joined a Junior Hockey team, he got serious about his equipment. One morning, I walked into the kitchen to see Justin draped over a burner, warming the blade of his hockey stick.

Me: *What are you doing?*

Justin: *Don't bother me, Mom. This is a two-hundred-dollar stick, and I'm heating the blade to give it a slight Right curve. If I mess it up, Dad won't be happy.*

Me: *I didn't know you could bend a wooden stick.*

Justin: *That's funny, Mom. Where've you been? Hockey sticks are made of carbon fibers, a strong and flexible material.*

Like heating the blade of a hockey stick to give it a curve, you will heat your strong and flexible ligaments to bend or straighten them.

RULE #6—A SPOT TO MOLD

This rule encourages you to find a comfortable place to mold. If your chosen spot has a **dual purpose,** your molding sessions will fit more readily into your schedule, and molding will become a habit.

Mold In Bed is the preferable place to mold, especially as you begin your Reverse Strategies. The advantage to molding in bed and under your covers is that it provides the warmth your muscles and ligaments need to help you relax and sink deeply into the molding stretch. Still, molding in bed serves an even greater purpose—it can help make molding a habit, and it goes something like this…

Everyone, at some point in their day, climbs into bed with the intention of going to sleep and wakes up STILL in bed. If you mold right after climbing into bed (at night) and AGAIN right before getting out of bed (in the morning), you increase the probability of a molding routine. This recommendation really works, and the best part about molding in bed—you don't have to battle with your busy daytime schedule to find the time.

A word of warning: molding in your cozy, warm bed at nighttime may cause you to fall asleep on your device. Be aware it won't help to do more than 20 minutes, but it won't hurt the molding efforts either. If this happens to you, it's okay; sometime in the night, you will likely roll off the device. The only downside is that you may experience muscle soreness the next day.

A word of wisdom: set your alarm twenty minutes before you have to get up in the morning. When the alarm goes off, hit the snooze and grab your device. Sink deeply into the stretch and enjoy some awesome quiet time for meditation or prayer.

The dual purpose—mold and fall asleep or mold before the world gets up.

Shirley Finally Did It In Bed

One evening, Shirley stopped by my office, delighted to tell me she had just started her Reverse Strategies at home. I gave her a puzzled look because she was not a new patient. Shirley went on to explain that she would watch TV, fall asleep on the couch, and drag herself to bed in the wee hours of the morning. Feeling ashamed that this had been going on for the entire year, she admitted it was the reason she couldn't find time to mold. Suddenly, her eyes lit up excitedly.

"But guess what, Dr. Faith? I decided it was time to go to bed by nine p.m. and mold as soon as I slide under the covers. Now, I totally understand WHY you preach—mold in bed. You just want us to experience how easy and convenient it is, so it becomes a habit. I cannot even tell you how much I look forward to going to bed and nestling under my cozy covers with my neck over my Newdle and my low-back over my Twodle... you are one smaht Doc!"

Mold Over The Side Of Your Bed *(aka Gravity Monster Solution)* is the Reverse Strategy for *Bowling Ball Head–Pull Head Backward.* The recommendation is to lie WIDTH-WISE (side to side) on your bed. You should still be able to cover yourself with your blankets, and it's not too challenging for partners to orient themselves on opposite sides of the bed at the same time (it really does work). One of the benefits of hanging your head over the side of the bed is that you don't have to remove pillows. When you are finished molding, do a scootch and half-turn, and you are right back at the top of your bed. For more support, lay the shorter Wedge piece under your shoulders so your head doesn't touch the bed. For more resistance, use the higher Wedge piece.

To offset gravity's constant pull, it is advised to "hang your head" over the side of your bed every night for the rest of your life. If you do nothing else but this strategy, this is the one. *Gravity Monster Solution is the... most... valuable... molding... stretch!* You don't need a device to hang your head over the side of your bed, and you don't need to wait until you've finished this book, either. Start right NOW.

The dual purpose—mold and thwart the gravity monster.

The Torture Chamber

Many patients told us they used their molding session as their quiet/meditation time. One woman shared that she tucked herself away in her walk-in closet, hung her head over a workout bench, and experienced some of the best alone time she'd ever had. Another woman took her work breaks, lying over her devices on the floor of an empty cubicle. An older gentleman told us he molded over the back of a lawn chair while being serenaded by birds outside his screened-in porch.

In our office, we had an entire room dedicated to molding. We heated it to eighty-five degrees, played soft music, and enforced a "quiet policy." Despite us calling it the molding room, most people jokingly referred to it as "the torture chamber." It was the most LOVED and HATED room in our office. As you'll soon find out, the Reverse Strategies can feel a bit torturous initially; that's the ***hate part***. As you put more time and effort into getting past the Elastic Phase and into the Plastic Phase, your body will like it and then crave it; that's the ***love part*** (I promise this to be true).

Allow me to clarify: recall that the natural curvy alignment of the neck bones is also the natural alignment for the brainstem and spinal cord (encased within the neck bones). That means, when a molding device gently pushes the neck into the Master Curve, feel-good beta-endorphins are released that promote whole-body calmness and that is addictive.

By the way: if you wake up during the night and can't get back to sleep, toss your pillow aside and grab your neck molding device. Your nervous system will relax, and your dream state will soon follow.

The dual purpose—mold to relax or mold to get back to sleep.

Mold On The Floor is probably the BETTER spot because it offers more resistance than the bed. Patients confirmed this over and over again but stressed how they ONLY moved to the floor when they were ready to *increase the push.* When you make it to the floor, you might listen to a podcast or TV show, *but be forewarned*: children and pets can make your attempts to mold on the floor almost IMPOSSIBLE. Inevitably, as you lay over a device, your son or daughter, pup or kitty is bound to think you want to play because you're at their level. Best of luck as you try to ward them off, or here's an idea for the kids, give THEM a device so they can mold with you.

The dual purpose—mold and learn or mold with your children.

Mold In The Bathroom (aka Bathroom Stretch) is the Reverse Strategy for a *Quirky Twisted* and *Tilted Head* and a *Quirky Shoulder*. It's a *hold that molding stretch* combined with muscle tension for 5 slow breaths in and out of the nose, 3x/day. Since you visit the bathroom multiple times a day, it makes the perfect private spot to close your eyes, concentrate on the stretch, hold, tense, and breathe your *Quirky's* away. Place a sticky note on your bathroom mirror to remind you to do your stretch every time you visit the bathroom. This "spot to mold" could be considered *Quirky*, but it's effective!

The dual purpose—pee first, then mold.

Implementing the Reverse Strategies into your daily schedule will take a fair amount of commitment and effort. Patients who had the most success molding beyond their second year were those who found a *regularly scheduled time* and a *designated place* to mold. Remember, Carol put her closet to use while the kids were at school, Janice used her cubicle at lunch, and Max molded on his porch after coffee. Get creative with your "molding spots" and work the stretches into the nooks and crannies of your day, or enjoy the *before and after* bedtime routine. Molding shouldn't be something you dread doing, like a chore, but more like brushing your teeth regularly, a very good habit.

RULE #7—STEADILY INCREASE THE PUSH

The Reverse Strategies work like making JELLO and remind me of my Great-Aunt Tillie's famous orange ambrosia. Solidified in a glass bowl with wavy edges, she would flop that jello salad out of the bowl onto a platter to be served with dinner. Not only was it a beautifully shaped piece of art, but it was also the best-tasting part of our Sunday meal!

Similarly, orthopedic devices are the "molding bowls" that will reshape your faulty parts. Rule #2 recommends five different-shaped devices with varying sizes for you to choose from to ACT as your "molding bowl."

Q: *How will you decide which devices will work for you?*

A: What is REALLY important is that whatever shape and size you use, it MUST *steadily increase the push* on the target site.

To *steadily increase the push* means your device must be adequately shaped and sized so that you feel it pushing on the faulty part when you lay over it. If you feel slightly uncomfortable, it's all right, but if you can't bear it right from the start, DOWN-SIZE the device height. If you're not feeling enough pressure at the target site, UP-SIZE the device height.

For example, you begin molding your neck with the **2-inch Newdle**, but it's too comfortable. You up-size to the **2 1/2 inch Newdle**, but it's still too easy. Your choices would be to try the **2 3/4 inch Newdle or Twodle** and maybe use a folded washcloth UNDER the device for increased height OR up-size to the Tower, but **PLEASE DO NOT USE** the **3 1/4 inch Twodle** nor **Half** or **Full Moon** under your neck.

Here's the reason for this cautionary measure: neck devices should ONLY push on the neck bones. If the device's height is too wide (fat), it will push on the skull, which should be avoided because the skull isn't the target site. Many types of neck devices are available to purchase online, but most are **too wide** for the neck, and that's why I can't endorse them. The exception to this rule is for long and large people.

Each strategy's device recommendations were made for the average-sized person. If you have long and/or large skeletal parts, you will have to make adjustments accordingly. If your structure allows you to use a **3 1/4 inch Twodle** under your neck, and it fits well, meaning your skull doesn't rest on the device, it's okay to use. I've had very large men handle the **4-inch Moon** under their lower-back without a problem, but if I used it there, it would send me to the MOON!

Pushing Force Rule Of Thumb

This *rule of thumb* is practical advice for the molding process, and it goes like this:

> *IF YOU DON'T FEEL THE DEVICE PUSHING ON THE FAULTY PART, LIGAMENTS WON'T CREEP/ STRETCH, AND BONES WON'T SHIFT AND STAY.*

Don't waste your molding sessions; keep up-sizing the device height, stack a book or two underneath, or use any gadget you can think of to *increase the push* on the target site.

RULE #8—CAUTION

As you begin molding, you'll find out fairly quickly that the areas being pushed and shoved become tender and sore. That's normal and relatively *short-term* because it will eventually subside. Having said that, there's something else you should be aware of that's relatively *long-term*. Because the molding stretches intentionally disrupt soft tissue fibers, they are *vulnerable to injury.*

It's entirely possible that one day you'll reach above your head to grab something out of the cabinet, bend over to pick up a toy, or twist and extend to reach into the back seat of the car, and suddenly the muscles, tendons, and ligaments you've been molding, are stretched beyond their comfort. Essentially, you've" tweaked" the soft tissue. It's not the end of the world, but it can feel like your old condition has returned. If this happens to you, take a molding break (Rule #4) and be cautious of putting yourself in compromised positions thereafter.

RULE #9—A SLOW AND STEADY FREQUENCY

Molding ANY faulty part to reshape into a curve or make them straight means the ligaments were stretched, and the bones conformed to a curvy or straightened position. It won't happen overnight, but you will be on your way to making it happen when you can easily and comfortably mold EACH Reverse Strategy for 20 minutes straight (in a single session). This rule is here to help you reach the 20-minute mark by encouraging you to take a slow and steady pace. Begin by molding 2-3 faulty parts EVERY DAY, and rotate your strategies. Recall that it's more important to mold for 5 minutes, get good and comfortable, then **slowly and steadily** work toward 20 minutes. A "slow and steady frequency" has many benefits:

- It will allow your body to get used to being pushed and pulled every day.
- It will help you avoid molding ALL your strategies EVERY DAY (a molding pace that's more like a race).
- It will ensure you focus on reversing ALL your faulty skeletal parts, not just one or two.

To help you track a steady pace, this rule recommends keeping a journal. *Do you have a used "subject" notebook lying around?* It might seem antiquated, but you can repurpose them and track your molding journey more successfully than mental memory. The nice thing about using a notebook is that you can write dates and memos daily, weekly, or anytime. Keep it simple and log strategies and molding minutes, or add more detail and jot down how you are *feeling and functioning.* Journaling is a great way to help support a slow and steady molding routine.

Earl's Exaggerated Presentation

When Earl walked into our office, I'll admit it—I was scared. It was early in my career, and I had never seen such an exaggerated "presentation," so I doubted how effective the Reverse Strategies would be.

Earl had been an egg farmer all his life and, at the age of seventy, still eagerly helped his sons with farming duties. Earl complained that his low-back and legs would get weak and painful mid-morning, which forced him to return to his house, get off his feet, and take a nap. After lunch, he'd return to the barn for a couple of hours before his low-back and legs would force him home again. Earl's **Structural Evaluation** revealed his "type" was *Boobs Meet Belly.* His low-back **pre-X-ray** confirmed an All-Shift-Together Misalignment complicated by Shift-And-Separate Misalignments. **See pages 15 and 16, images 2B, 2D**.

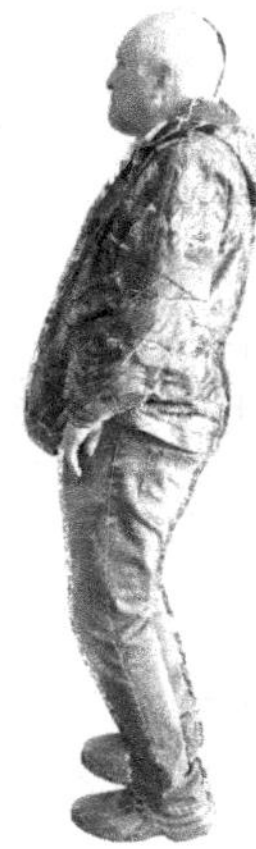

When Earl began his Reverse Strategies, he could only mold his low-back curve for a minute at a time. Molding up to 6x daily, he steadily increased those minutes. At three months, Earl moved his molding routine from his bed onto the floor. At six months, Earl reported with excitement that he had more energy, needed only a single break for lunch, and worked the entire day without his usual low-back and leg pain. At twelve months, we took a **post-X-ray**, and as you can see, there was a huge improvement!

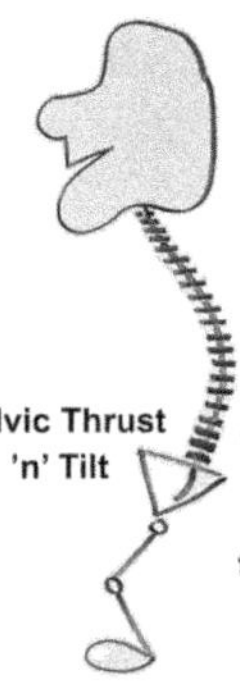

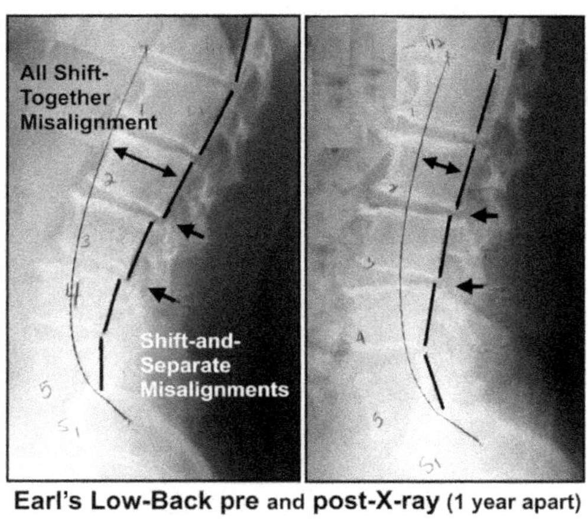

Earl's Low-Back pre and post-X-ray (1 year apart)

RULE #10—DOUBLE WHAMMY

This rule means you can double your efforts by molding two faulty parts simultaneously to save time. Make sure you are plenty comfortable with your strategies BEFORE you attempt to double up. Double Whammy is recommended for those who can mold for 5 minutes straight. Try these molding pairs: restore neck and low-back curves, restore middle-back and sacrum curves, *Gravity Monster Solution* and reverse *HunchBack Shoulders*, reverse *HunchBack Shoulders* and restore neck curve. Double Whammy is a time management idea that can help you fit ALL your Reverse Strategies into your weekly schedule. The charts listed below can further assist you.

RULE #11—MAKE A MOLDING PLAN

When you "make a molding plan," you set "the goal" in motion, and your first goal should be to mold **each** Reverse Strategy for 20 minutes STRAIGHT (one session). This rule encourages you to organize your Reverse Strategies into a daily and weekly schedule to move towards that goal. To guide you, use the pre-formatted molding schedule for YOUR Bad Back Type and modify it as you see fit. Remember, how often you mold and how many strategies you mold in a single day should always support your own pace.

Each schedule has been formatted into a six-day cycle to include a morning and bedtime routine. The expectation is that you will mold for six days, take the seventh day off, and mold in bed. Additionally, *Quirky's* have been included with each schedule.

Molding Phases (Step 10) can give you more information to help you reach your molding goals. To print your Molding Schedule, go to our website.

FRONT LOADER **Reverse Strategy (#1, #2, #4) Molding Schedule (Refer to Steps 7, 8, 10)**	
Follow Column 1 and Mold on Days: 1, 3, 5	**Follow Column 2 and Mold on Days: 2, 4, 6**
Mold the Reverse Strategies listed in the row below before getting out of bed (A.M.)	
(#2) Reverse **Cold Shoulders —>** (Part I) Push Them Backward 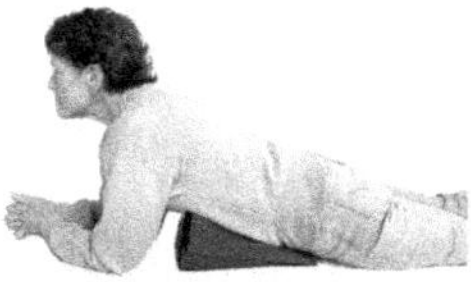	(#4) Reverse **Pelvic Thrust 'n' Tilt —>** (Part I) Push Pelvis Backward 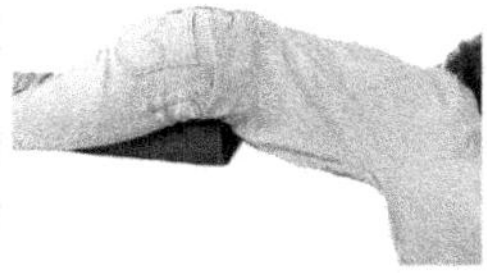
Mold the Reverse Strategies listed in the row below immediately upon climbing into bed (P.M.)	
(#1) Reverse **Bowling** Ball **Head** (Part I) —> Pull Head Backward ***(aka Gravity Monster Solution)*** 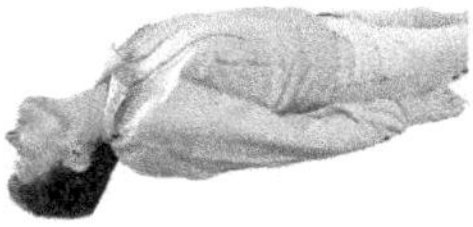	(#1) Reverse **Bowling Ball Head** (Part II) —> Push Neck Forward 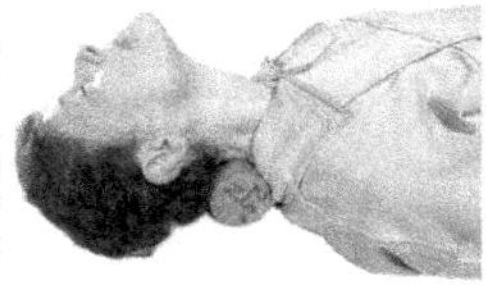
Mold the Reverse Strategies listed in the row below directly after the above strategy (P.M.)	
(#4) Reverse **Pelvic Thrust 'n' Tilt —>** (Part II) Push Sacrum Forward 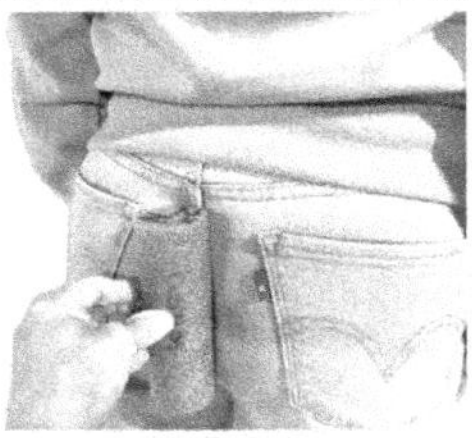 ~ (#2) Reverse **Cold Shoulders** (Part II) —> Push Middle-Back Forward 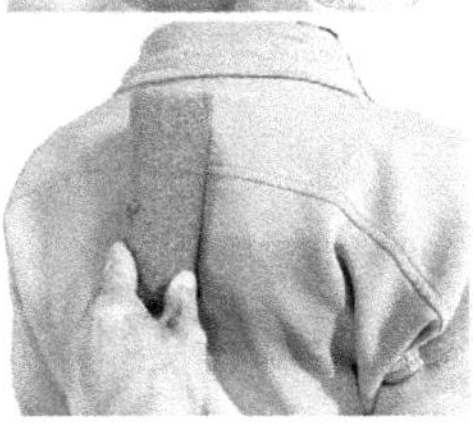	(#4) Reverse **Pelvic Thrust 'n' Tilt —>** (Part III) Push Low-Back Forward 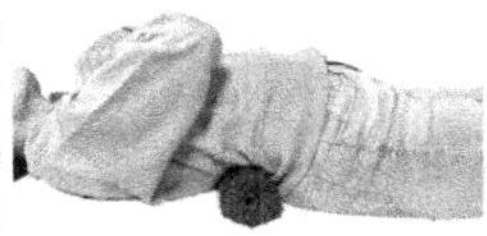
Mold the *Quirky's* listed in the row below ANYTIME during your day (Refer to Step 7, 8, 10)	
Reverse ***Quirky* Sideways Head —>** To reverse a ***Quirky* Twisted**, and **Tilted Head,** and a ***Quirky* Shoulder**. Use the Bathroom Stretch found in Step 8, Rule #6. Push Head Opposite 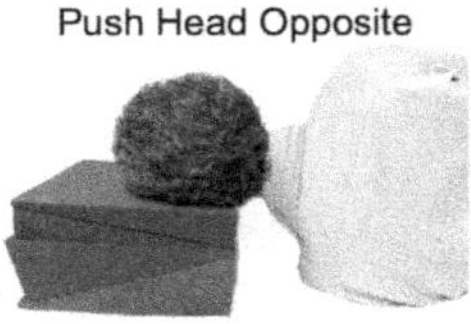	Reverse ***Quirky* Pelvis —>** Push Pelvis Opposite 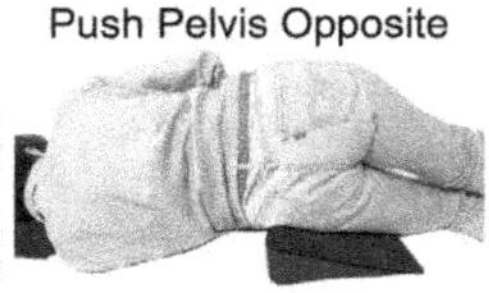
Column 1	**Column 2**

BOOBS MEET BELLY **Reverse Strategy (#1, #3, #4) Molding Schedule (Refer to Steps 7, 8, 10)**	
Follow Column 1 and Mold on Days: 1, 3, 5	**Follow Column 2 and Mold on Days: 2, 4, 6**
Mold the Reverse Strategies listed in the row below before getting out of bed (A.M.)	
(#3) Reverse **Hunchback Shoulders** (Part I) —> Push Them Forward 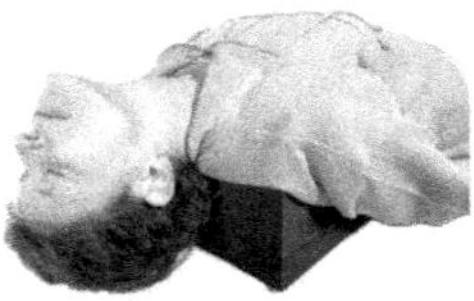	(#4) Reverse **Pelvic Thrust 'n' Tilt —>** (Part I) Push Pelvis Backward 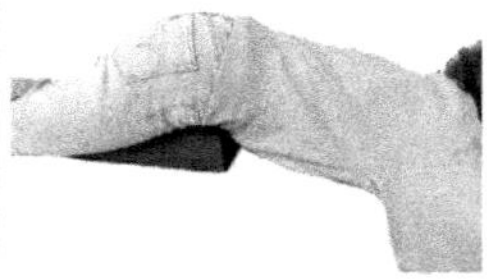
Mold the Reverse Strategies listed in the row below immediately upon climbing into bed (P.M.)	
(#1) Reverse **Bowling** Ball **Head** (Part I) —> Pull Head Backward ***(aka Gravity Monster Solution)*** 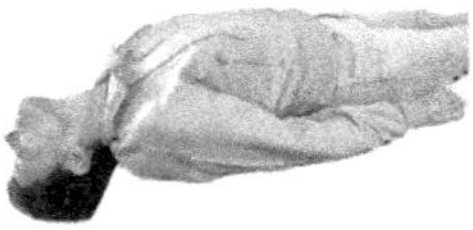	(#1) Reverse **Bowling Ball Head** (Part II) —> Push Neck Forward 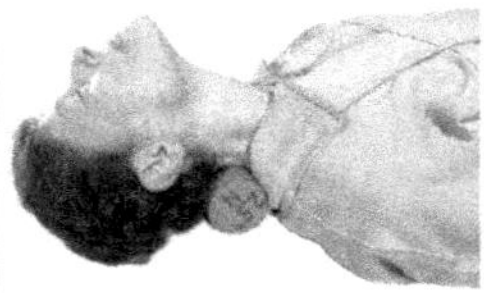
Mold the Reverse Strategies listed in the row below directly after the above strategy (P.M.)	
(#4) Reverse **Pelvic Thrust 'n' Tilt —>** (Part II) Push Sacrum Forward 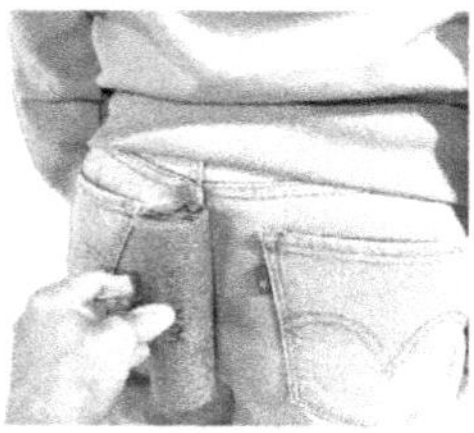 ~ (#2) Reverse **Cold Shoulders** (Part II) —> Push Middle-Back Forward (optional for BMB types) 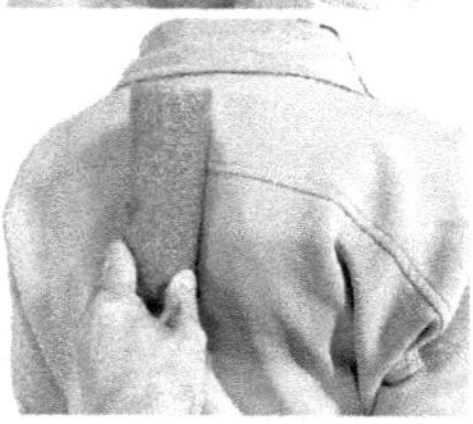	(#4) Reverse **Pelvic Thrust 'n' Tilt —>** (Part III) Push Low-Back Forward 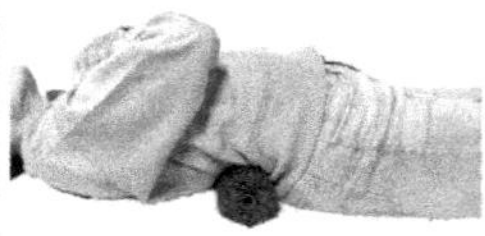
Mold the *Quirky's* listed in the row below ANYTIME during your day (Refer to Step 7, 8, 10)	
Reverse ***Quirky*** **Sideways Head —>** Push Head Opposite 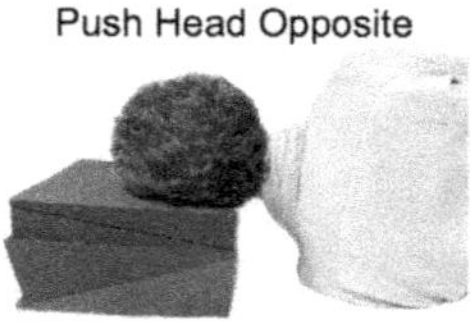 To reverse a ***Quirky*** **Twisted**, and **Tilted Head**, and a ***Quirky*** **Shoulder**. Use the Bathroom Stretch found in Step 8, Rule #6.	Reverse ***Quirky*** **Pelvis —>** Push Pelvis Opposite 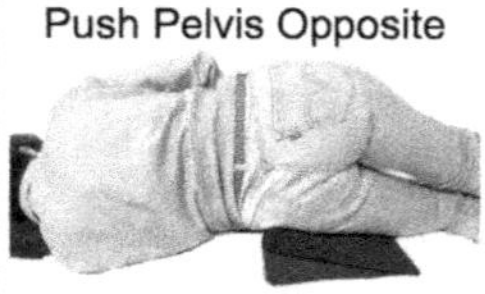
Column 1	**Column 2**

THE STOOP **Reverse Strategy (#1, #2, #5) Molding Schedule (Refer to Steps 7, 8, 10)**	
Follow Column 1 and Mold on Days: 1, 3, 5	**Follow Column 2 and Mold on Days: 2, 4, 6**
Mold the Reverse Strategies listed in the row below before getting out of bed (A.M.)	
(#2) Reverse **Cold Shoulders —>** (Part I) Push Them Backward 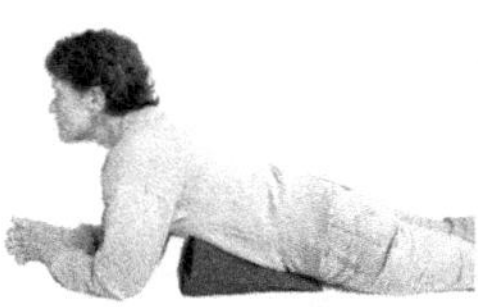	(#5) Reverse **Pelvic Back-Ender w/ Dip** —> (Part I) Push Pelvis Forward 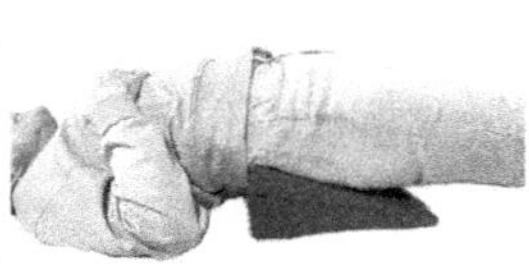
Mold the Reverse Strategies listed in the row below immediately upon climbing into bed (P.M.)	
(#1) Reverse **Bowling Ball Head** (Part I) **—>** Pull Head Backward ***(aka Gravity Monster Solution)*** 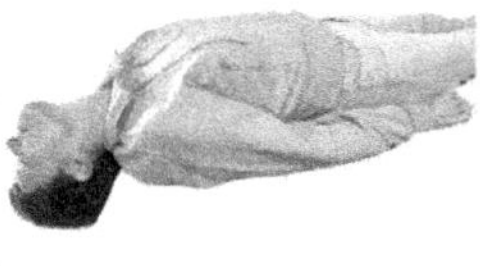	(#1) Reverse **Bowling Ball Head** (Part II) **—>** Push Neck Forward 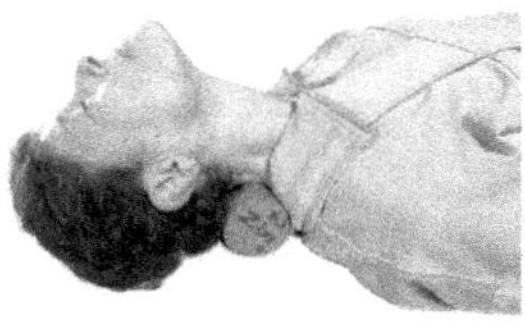
Mold the Reverse Strategies listed in the row below directly after the above strategy (P.M.)	
(#2) Reverse **Cold Shoulders —>** (Part II) Push Middle-Back Forward 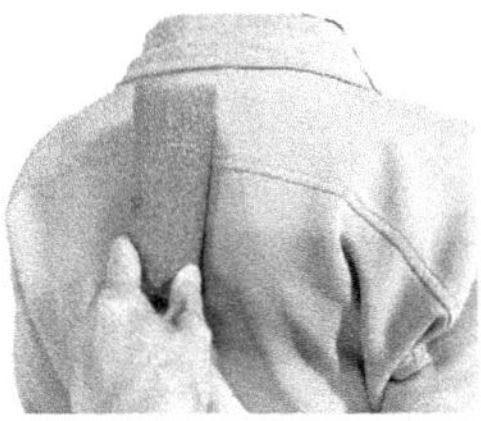	(#5) Reverse **Pelvic Back-Ender w/ Dip —>** (Part II) Push Low-Back Forward 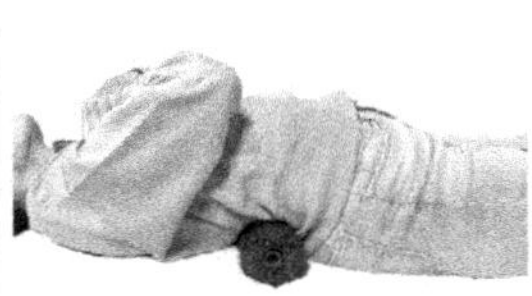
Mold the *Quirky's* listed in the row below ANYTIME during your day (Refer to Step 7, 8, 10)	
Reverse ***Quirky* Sideways Head —>** To reverse a ***Quirky* Twisted**, and **Tilted Head**, and a ***Quirky* Shoulder**. Use the Bathroom Stretch found in Step 8, Rule #6. Push Head Opposite 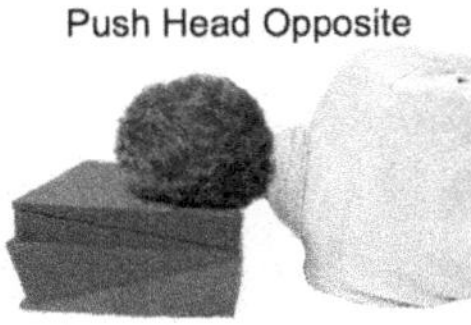	Reverse ***Quirky* Pelvis —>** Push Pelvis Opposite 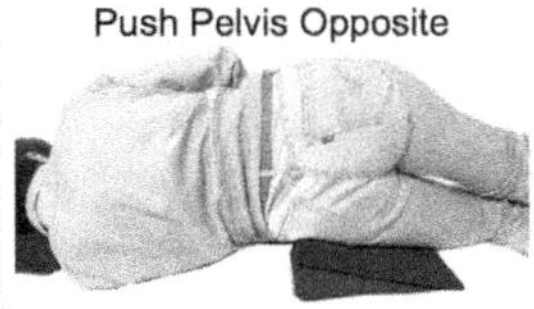
Column 1	**Column 2**

RULE #12—MAKE YOUR STRATEGIES ROUTINE

This rule asks you to be honest with yourself. *Can you make molding part of your life?* Although you've been taught to mold while watching TV, taking a work break, and sleeping, the truth is that molding until your back problems are permanently resolved is going to require a fair amount of **commitment**.

For years, Mom would wait until I was already cozy in my bed. She would march upstairs so I could hear every footstep, enter my bedroom, and lean in so we were cheek to cheek. She would smell my breath and then, in a whisper, ask, *"Did you brush your teeth?"* Of course, already privy to the answer, she would watch me reluctantly get out of bed and stand in the bathroom doorway to ensure I brushed. It didn't take me long to make brushing my teeth BEFORE I climbed into bed a nightly routine, and since then, I've never gone to bed without brushing.

Similarly, *why go to bed without molding?* Although molding isn't as easy as brushing and flossing, without making a commitment to a daily routine, your back will ROT, just like your teeth!

RULE #13—BE AFRAID

Like Friday the 13th, you and the entire human race should be afraid of Rule #13. It warns us of our INTENSE screen usage. Screens are pulling our skeletal structures downward with more force than gravity. This rule asks us to look around at the seniors who are bent and contorted and moving closer to the ground every day because gravity has already worked its law on their bones. **See page 162, image 10B**.

Let this rule be a warning: unless you take the steps to reverse your Bad Back Type, your skeletal structure will degrade well before its time. Learn and implement the Reverse Strategies into your daily schedule. Pass this method along to your family and friends, and trust that it will keep us ALL upright, tall, straight, and proud with our heads held high for years to come.

Part IV

KEEP UP TO JOIN UP

STEP 9: APPLY THE GOOD BACK HABITS

My Breakthrough

It all started when we opened our second office in a new location, several states away. To get the practice off the ground, we ran a "Grand Opening Special" with the local Groupon®, promoting a Structural Evaluation and Massage for $20. It was Friday at noon when the ad went "live," and the phone began to ring off the hook. Sarah, my assistant, gave me a *here we go* glance and picked up the phone to schedule the first of the one hundred recipients who took us up on our offer. Our Massage Therapist was available on Saturdays, so the next morning, they began to arrive.

Debbie sat quietly, reading the brochure I gave her while I studied the complaints on her intake form. As I pointed out Johnny's Bad Back Signs, she watched attentively. Then, she stood excitedly in front of the mirror for her Structural Evaluation, staring at her head and shoulders.

Debbie: *Wow, my Right shoulder is much lower than my Left, and my head definitely leans in that direction. Are you sure my backbone is responsible for this, or is it because I've sat at a desk for nearly thirty years?*

Me: *Yes, both. Your head and shoulders suggest your backbone shifted. Without an accident to blame, this probably occurred over the course of your career. Now, those faulty parts are likely the reason you get tension headaches, shoulder pain, and tingling in your Right hand.*

Over and over, for six solid months, I reviewed complaints and evaluated the skeletal structures of **every... voucher... holder**. Truth be told, none of these people sought our office for back pain and problems (they just wanted a $20 massage), but after being evaluated, most WANTED to address their Bad Back. For those interested, I invited them to our new patient class, *The Real Reason Your Back Hurts*, and offered a FREE set of X-rays if they attended. It was a huge success; our classes were always full, and our practice grew.

To accommodate the growing number of patients, we had to create a second class, *Take Your Bad Back and Make it a Good Back,* to teach the Reverse Strategies (that's when I "fit" patients with their orthopedic devices). Shortly after, we developed a third class, *The Good Back Habits*, to address the ongoing inquiries related to mattresses, pillows, shoes, standing, walking, and more. To my surprise, the class was remarkably popular and well-attended. I thought it was because the topics addressed common, everyday stuff, but that wasn't the feedback I received. Patients unanimously agreed that applying *The Good Back Habits* supported their lifestyle in ways they hadn't expected. Here are a few testimonials:

> *"Learning how to correctly stand, sit, and walk made me very aware of my sloppy habits and how they supported my OLD pattern. Now, I am constantly correcting myself because good habits just feel good."*

> *"I brought my husband to the workshop, and we both felt immediate improvements when we began practicing EVERYTHING Dr. Faith recommended. You can't get this information anywhere; it's like a treasure chest!"*

> *"Every single habit is a lifestyle change for the better, and like "icing on the cake," they ALL enhance the Reverse Strategies."*

I love positive feedback and am always grateful for the ideas that emerge from them. Shortly after reading Cheryl's "treasure chest" comment, I began jotting down information from these classes, which inspired the writing of this book.

THE GOOD BACK HABITS

The Good Back Habits are **only** designed to support the Reverse Strategies, so please DO NOT expect them to make your Bad Back a Good Back **all on their own**. However, if you incorporate these habits into your lifestyle, making your Bad Back good is guaranteed to be easier and faster.

- **Activity-Based Habits:** Standing, Walking, Stretching
- **Resting-Based Habits:** Sitting, Sleeping
- **Recovery-Based Habits:** Soft Tissue Therapy, Foot Therapy, Backbone Therapy

ACTIVITY-BASED STANDING HABITS

Stand At Attention Habit

To "stand at attention," I want you to stand up, place your hands on your waist, and **roll** your pelvis forward (this is NOT a push; it's a rotation). To roll the pelvis forward, use your thumbs to push the low-back forward while using your fingers to push the hips backward until your low-back aches (if it doesn't ache, roll harder).

Next, hold the pelvis in this rolled forward position by pushing your low-back curve into your stomach (allow your stomach to bulge). Then, raise your upper body until your shoulders hover over your hips and heels (they should ALL line up). Lastly, keep the curve but relax the stomach muscles. If you are standing correctly, all your weight will be on your heels, so your toes might come up off the floor.

When you "stand at attention," you are standing in *The Good Back Type*, so you will look good, and it's an "energizing pose," so you will feel good. Best of all, it can help you **avoid** pushing the pelvis. The next time you stand in conversation or in line at the grocery store, ROLL (your pelvis), PUSH (your curve), and LINE-UP (your shoulders, hips, and heels).

Bear in mind: your pelvis will RELAX, and this standing pose will become slouchy when you stop concentrating on standing correctly. When you catch yourself slouching, remember to **do... this... one... thing...** PUSH YOUR LOW-BACK CURVE INTO YOUR STOMACH. This "one thing" will help you remember to "stand at attention," and once again, you'll be supporting a Good Back!

The Guilty Party

When you "stand at attention," you will undoubtedly feel like you're flaunting your chest and buttocks. Yep, it doesn't feel natural at all, but it definitely looks GOOD (assume the pose and ask someone). The reality is that every time you "stand at attention," your pelvis lines up with your upper and lower body, which makes it... **center-aligned**.

You MUST practice "stand at attention" as often as possible until holding your pelvis in that **rolled forward position** becomes **natural**. If you don't, you'll continue to push your pelvis into its old pelvic pattern, which reinforces your old Bad Back Type. STOP PUSHING your pelvis and understand THAT IS EXACTLY how your "type" developed in the first place. It all started when your pelvis pushed forward or backward, and your upper body HAD to shift in the opposite direction.

Remember when I said it's the backbone's fault in Step 1? Well, the truth is, the pelvis is *the guilty party*, and it's responsible for your Bad Back Type. If you want to put an END to your pushing pelvis, keep *the guilty party* center-aligned and "stand at attention" **all... the... time!**

Tree Trunk Habit

For "tree trunk," I want you to stand up with your legs and feet together (as tight as possible) or keep your heels together and toes apart, like a "V." Now, tense (squeeze) your butt cheeks, thighs, and legs. Hold a medium tension, think, *I'm sturdy like an oak tree,* and don't forget to breathe.

Tree Trunk can be used when standing STILL, like in conversation in line at the airport. Tree Trunk your lower body **first** so it's firmly anchored (keep the tension), then "stand at attention." This DUO may deter you from *wanting* to lean on a chair, counter, or wall (like you are bored), throwing your leg out to the side (like you are cool), or sitting on one of your hips (like it's supporting a baby). Those slouchy standing habits make you look sloppy and **encourage** the pelvis to push, which encourages a Bad Back. Instead, combine "tree trunk" with "stand at attention" to look amazing and feel energized!

Additionally, Tree Trunk can be used when standing HUNCHED OVER a task. This pose supports the upper body but doesn't compromise the lower parts of the backbone or pelvis. So, let's say you are hunched over the counter chopping vegetables or over the stove sautéing dinner; Tree Trunk your lower body **first**, then lean over your task.

When I began practicing this habit, I wrote on a sticky note, TREE TRUNK, and put it above the sink. As I washed dishes, I could only hold this pose for about 30 seconds before I got tired, but the more I practiced, the longer I could hold it. This habit takes A LOT of practice and a good amount of concentration, and with persistence, you'll **avoid** pushing the pelvis as you stand to support the Good Back.

Paulette's Basket

Paulette was a lively 85-year-old woman who came for weekly office visits and brightened our day with her infectious, happy mood! After her Adjustment, she would sing this little song as she made her way to our molding room.... *See me walk so straight and tall; I won't let my basket fall... eyes ahead and don't look down; keep that basket off the ground.*

Let Paulette's jingle be a reminder that, into our elder years, we should STILL be standing upright, tall, straight, and proud with our heads held high!

Back Pocket Habit

This standing habit is designed for those who tend to cross their arms out in front of their body or put their hands in the front pockets of their pants or coats. If this is you, you are forcing your shoulders to fold down and in. Instead, place your hands in the pants' back pockets or clasp your hands (or forearms) together behind you. This habit reinforces the Reverse *Cold/HunchBack Shoulder* Strategy, makes *standing at attention* that much easier, and transforms your slouchy, worn-out look into an attentive and confident appearance!

Humans Must Stand Upright

The cosmic source of energy, Life Force, enters the human body at the back of the head between the skull and Atlas (neck bone #1). Life Force isn't visible to our naked eye or with any instrument because it's smaller than protons and electrons (imagine wind without hearing or feeling it). Life Force is spiritual energy, and it flows subtly alongside the physical energy of the nervous system to silently **activate** ALL bodily functions.

To obtain Life Force energy at its fullest, the backbone cannot be tilted, twisted, or bent sideways, and it certainly can't have straight, exaggerated, or reversed curves because those misalignments can diminish the flow of nerve energy and, therefore, Life Force energy. People with a low supply of Life Force have a depressed body, mind, and spirit. They are weak, frail, and sickly, and their skeletal structure depicts a Bad Back Type in an advanced phase. *Humans must stand upright*; our Life Force depends on it!

Pigeon—Toed

One of my earliest childhood memories dates back to a pair of leg braces I wore because I was severely pigeon-toed. According to my mother, I was born with inward-turned hips, and to rectify this, leg braces were recommended. I was two years old when I was fitted and wore the braces for two years. As the doctor removed them, I clearly remember him saying, *"Faith, concentrate on slowly placing each heel firmly on the ground with your foot straight, and don't let your foot toe in."*

When I got to middle school, it didn't take long to realize that I needed to concentrate harder on placing my feet straight ahead instead of toeing inward to avoid nasty, juvenile comments. It must have worked because my foot pattern in the snow shows ONLY a slight inward tendency. Being pigeon-toed didn't resolve itself entirely through my willful foot placement. Still, it gave me the personal experience and desire to spend countless hours analyzing the *activity of walking* to create what I believe is the "perfect walk."

ACTIVITY-BASED WALKING HABITS

Place-Tense-Wiggle Habit

When we walk, all 5 pelvic joints should engage in the activity, not just the 2 hip joints. **See Step 3, images 3D, 3E**. This walking habit ensures all 5 pelvic joints get involved, and it's BEST learned in 2 parts, but it's actually 3 separate actions. To begin, start walking across the room…

PART 1: Place (step) each foot so that your heel strikes the floor first, then roll onto your toes for a good "push-off." Walking should be a quiet, light-footed action, so **do not** let the ball of your foot hit first. Take several practice steps across the room and back with a stride that's comfortable enough to PLACE your heel first. Now add the TENSE…

PART 2: Tense is a butt cheek squeeze, **after** you've *placed*. So, *place* your Left foot, then TENSE (squeeze) your Left butt cheek. *Place* your Right foot, then TENSE your Right butt cheek. Take several practice steps across the room and back. Now add the WIGGLE…

Wiggle is an "intentional push" of your butt cheek to the side, at **exactly** the same moment as you *tense* (occurs simultaneously). So, *place* your Left foot, then *tense* your Left butt cheek as you WIGGLE (push) to the Right. *Place* your Right foot, then *tense* the Right butt cheek as you WIGGLE (push) to the Left.

Next, add in more GRIT and GRIND so that when you *tense* your butt cheek, you squeeze it harder, and when you *wiggle*, you use more force to "push" and dig into your hip joint. Now, practice *place—tense—wiggle* across the room and back a few times. If you are walking correctly, you should feel like a model walking down the runway. Although that slow pace is fine for learning to *walk this way*, a faster pace makes it easier to *tense—wiggle*, which provides the "oomph" necessary to *place* each foot.

Don't waste the opportunity to *place—tense—wiggle* to the bathroom, across the street, or through the park. Wherever you go, remember to **do… this… one… thing…** SQUEEZE YOUR BUTT CHEEK AS YOU PUSH IT. This "one thing" will help you remember to *walk this way*. When you include this habit into your lifestyle, you will be the **envy** of anyone who watches you walk. Practice continually, and you should notice your butt muscles becoming toned… *Is it possible a flat butt becomes rounder?* YES, but it will take a good amount of *grit and grind*, and you will have to walk like this **all… the… time!**

Walk Your Pelvis To Avoid A Hip Replacement

Walking **requires** the movement and flexibility of all 5 pelvic joints: two SI joints (sacroiliac), one L5-S1 joint (sacral base), and two hip joints (femur heads). When the pelvis is NO LONGER center-aligned (because of a thrust, back-ender, or *Quirky*), it causes an unequal distribution of weight among the 5 pelvic joints. The joints with the greater "load" will **jam** (usually the 2 hip joints), degenerate, and eventually need to be replaced. To avoid this scenario, reverse your pelvic "signs" to equalize the "load," then *place—tense—wiggle* wherever you go so ALL 5 pelvic joints get a good **workout**. *Walk your pelvis* because pelvic flexibility is the key to maintaining a Good Back.

PELVIC JOINTS THAT RUB AND CRACK is a condition that begins when there's an unequal distribution of weight among the 5 pelvic joints. As a person walks, the joints with more "load" rub together to produce a horrible cracking sound that's annoying and sometimes painful. When our patients (with this condition) reversed their pelvic "signs" and used *place—tense—wiggle*, the "rubbing and cracking" went away. When the load on weight-bearing joints becomes more equalized and the pelvic joints become more flexible, problems can resolve.

Supportive Walking Habits

If you are a fast-paced walker, road warrior, slow-paced jogger, or sidewalk mosey-er, you will appreciate a few tips to improve your efficiency while supporting a Good Back:

- Keep your upper body upright so it hovers over your pelvis. **Don't lean forward.**
- Keep your head held high so it looks ahead. **Don't look down at your feet.**
- Keep "placing" the heel of your foot so it hits the pavement first. **Don't be a ball slapper.**

GB—9 Sequence

This Good Back (GB) sequence of 9 standing stretches (4 back and 5 neck) energizes and tones muscles, ligaments, tendons, joints, and nerves. Combine the Tree Trunk Habit with these standing stretches to transform your experience. To print this sequence, go to our website.

ACTIVITY-BASED STRETCHING HABITS

1. **Backbone Tension**—Cross arms while holding opposite elbows. Tense and release butt cheeks, tense and release low-back (push into stomach), tense and release middle-back (push it backward), tense and release upper-back (shoulders and blades); that's one round. Repeat 3-5x.
2. **Backbone Twists**—Keep arms crossed. Twist (with force) upper body to the Left, twist (with force) upper body to the Right; that's one round. Repeat 5-10x.
3. **Backbone Side Bends**—Arms at side. Bend upper body to the Left, and bring the Right arm overhead, bend the upper body to the Right, and bring the Left arm overhead; that's one round. Repeat 5-10x.
4. **Front Bends**—Hands on waist. Bend upper body forward, bend backward; that's one round. Repeat 5-10x.
5. **Neck Side Bends**—Hands down at the side. Keep shoulders level. Bend Left ear to Left shoulder, bend Right ear to Right shoulder; that's one round. Repeat 3-5x.
6. **Neck Twists**—Twist neck Right, twist neck Left; that's one round. Repeat 3-5x.
7. **Neck Tension**—Keep the chin level. Tense and release Left neck muscles, tense and release Right neck muscles, tense and release throat muscles, tense and release back of neck muscles; that's one round. Repeat 2-3x.
8. **Neck Drop**—Drop the head (chin to chest). Tense ALL neck muscles, and hold that tension while S-L-O-W-L-Y pulling the head backward until the nose is pointing up at the ceiling, release tension; that's one round. Repeat 2-3x.
9. **Neck Roll**—Drop the head (chin to chest). S-l-o-w-l-y in a counterclockwise direction, roll neck all the way around; 2-3 times. S-l-o-w-l-y in a clockwise direction, roll neck all the way around; 2-3 times.

RESTING-BASED SITTING HABITS

Sit At Attention Habit

To "sit at attention," I want you to sit on a dining room chair or one with a backrest. Sit with your feet firmly on the floor. Lean your upper body forward so you can shimmy each butt cheek backward (butt back) until it's **squished tightly** against the back of the chair, and it can't go back any further. Still leaning, roll your pelvis forward by pushing your low-back curve into your stomach (allow your stomach to **bulge**), then raise your upper body until your shoulders rest against the backrest. Lastly, keep the curve, but relax your stomach muscles. If you are sitting correctly, you are likely thinking, *I've never actually sat this far back on any chair, but it really feels good!*

You can "sit at attention" just as easily on a stool, bench, or picnic table, and I promise you'll look better than the person sitting next to you. Still, you'll need to be *aware of the slouch:* your pelvis will RELAX, and you will slouch the moment you stop concentrating on sitting correctly. When you catch yourself slouching, remember to **do… this… one… thing…** PUSH YOUR LOW-BACK CURVE INTO YOUR STOMACH. This "one thing" will help you remember to "sit at attention," and once again, you'll be supporting a Good Back.

Sitting To Meditate

This recommendation addresses "how to" meditate while sitting, which reinforces the "sit at attention" habit. It caters to the growing number of people who are actively meditating and were taught to do so by sitting with their legs crossed in *Easy Pose.* If you want to learn how to meditate successfully, I wouldn't recommend sitting in *Easy Pose* on the floor, on a bed, on a cushion, or anywhere else. With your help, I'll prove there's a better way to meditate.

Begin by sitting on the floor with your legs crossed and hands gripping your kneecaps. Roll your pelvis forward and "sit at attention" (as I've instructed). This is *Easy Pose.* Now, close your eyes, and s-l-o-w-l-y breathe through your nose. *Could you hold this pose for twenty minutes or more without slouching*? Probably not. A slouchy back traps Life Force energy in the lowest parts of the backbone, so all efforts to get the body to BE STILL are overridden by bodily sensations of discomfort. Then, sitting for more than a few minutes becomes nearly impossible and certainly not long enough to establish "stillness of the mind."

An alternative to *Easy Pose* is *Lotus Pose.* Meditating yogis sit in this pretzel-like pose for hours because their intertwined legs and feet lock their pelvis, exactly like "sit at attention." When the pelvis is LOCKED in the rolled forward position, the backbone automatically straightens up. According to Patanjali (Eightfold Path of Yoga), successful meditation is **completely dependent** on the backbone being upright and straight. That's when Life Force can be drawn upward from the base of the pelvis, bodily sensations are nulled, and the yogi can sit… for… a… long… time to achieve "stillness of the mind."

If your body is flexible enough to sit in *Lotus Pose*, good golly, go for it, but *there's a better way to meditate:* Find a quiet spot, sit on a solid bench or chair (not against the backrest), place feet firmly on the floor and hands on the thighs (palms up). Sit At Attention (think Buddha Belly), set your gaze at the brow, and don't forget the earplugs!

Supportive Sitting Habits

- Sit in your chair with your butt pushed as far back as it will go. Sitting **"butt back"** can help you avoid the tendency to slouch.
- When sitting at a table or desk push your chair in as far as possible. This will reduce your need to lean forward and slouch.
- Cross your ankles instead of crossing your legs. This reduces strain on the SI joints.
- Get up from your office chair every twenty minutes or so for 2-3 minutes (set a timer). Take a short walk, use the restroom, or stretch. The longer you sit, the more likely you are to slouch.

- Sturdy-framed chairs, such as rocking chairs and dining room chairs, make "sitting at attention" very easy. They also make great office chairs.
- Support your low-back with a pillow or Newdle when sitting on a couch, recliner, or plush chair. These types of furniture are designed to be comfortable but encourage "sloppy" sitting.
- Take frequent TV breaks and do something active. Play with the kids, wrestle with the dog, load the dishwasher, or take out the trash. Lounging in a slouch for an extended period is undoing your Reverse Strategy efforts.

Daisy Duke Habit

As a teenager, I watched Daisy Duke strut her stuff every Friday night. It was weekly entertainment that I rarely missed. She was a kind and beautiful southern girl, and I downright loved her smile, short-shorts, and long legs, so I named this sitting habit after her. The Daisy Duke is how to get IN and OUT of any vehicle as a passenger or driver. Now, we all know that Daisy never swung her legs through the window of the *General Lee* to get inside (like Bo and Luke), but for the sake of this habit, *imagine this scenario:*

Daisy opens the *General Lee's* driver-side door, sits her butt down on the seat, then swings her legs around until they land inside the car. That's it. That's exactly how I would recommend you get into YOUR car. Exit similarly by sliding the seat backward (so you have room to get out), swinging your legs out the door, and firmly placing both feet on the ground to stand up.

Supportive Vehicle Sitting Habits

- Adjust the backrest so it's upright. A reclined backrest will increase stress on the low-back bones.
- Slide the seat forward until your foot generously rests on the gas pedal. Toe driving will stress the hip and SI joints.
- Sit on the seat, **"butt back"** to reduce low-back stress.
- Adjust the mirrors AFTER you sit *butt back*. If you notice you can't see out the rearview mirror during your ride, you have probably slumped.
- Adjust the headrest or reverse the headrest orientation so it doesn't push your head forward.
- Inflate the lumbar support to the maximum or put a Newdle behind your low-back to support the curve.
- Heated seats promote inflammation; turn them **off** after 10 minutes.
- As a passenger, use a travel pillow to help support your neck curve.

RESTING-BASED SLEEPING HABITS

Sleep Flat On Your Back Habit

The best position to sleep is "flat on your back" with NO pillow under your head. This position easily supports a vertically straight backbone. If you can't do without a pillow, use a very flat or feather pillow under your head and neck ONLY (not under shoulders). Fat, fluffy pillows are not recommended because they force the head and neck to tilt forward and encourage *Bowling Ball Head.*

Sleeping With Someone Who Snores

Why does my husband snore? This was a question I received so often that I began addressing the condition during our Reverse Strategy Class. The discussion began by showing this image of the hard and soft anatomy of the neck and throat.

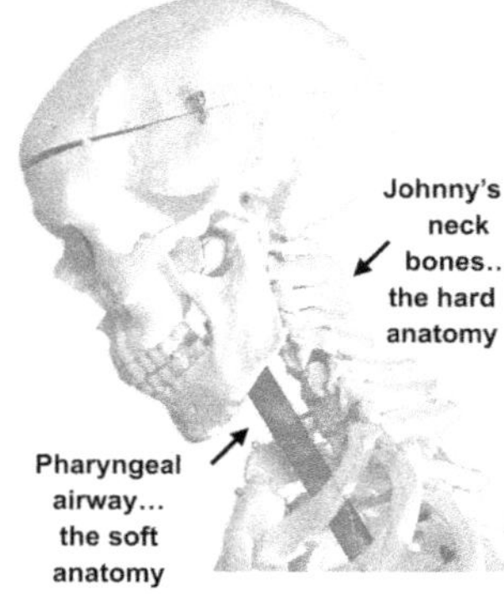

Then I'd explain that when the pharyngeal airway narrows and breathing becomes restricted, snoring is likely. That's when the wife tries to get her husband to roll onto his side, hoping this will correct the situation. With a quick review of the anatomy, we will see if her technique is the solution.

Q: *What lies directly behind the soft anatomy of the pharyngeal airway that could cause enough physical pressure to narrow the canal?*

A: The hard anatomy of the neck bones.

Bowling Ball Head causes the head to shift forward, and the neck bones follow. The more forward they shift, the greater the pressure on the pharyngeal airway. While the husband lies on his pillow at night (on his back), the physical stress of the neck bones on the airway will double because his pillow pushes his head and neck even more forward. If the wife rolls her husband onto his side, this should alleviate his snoring, which makes her technique a good solution.

If the wife wants her husband to STOP snoring, she will have to recommend he make *Reverse Bowling Ball Head Strategy* a part of his bedtime routine. These molding stretches will teach the hard neck bones to shift backward so they stop pushing on the soft airway.

Be forewarned: if the snorer falls asleep while molding the neck, the snoring is likely to get intense; bear with it. Snoring should slowly reduce and hopefully disappear altogether.

Supportive Sleeping Habits

- Stomach sleeping forces the head to twist. This is the most common reason for a *Quirky Twisted Head*. If you must, keep your head centered and rest your chin on the mattress.
- Tilt your head upward when sleeping on your side; NEVER tilt downward.
- Side sleeping on a fat, fluffy pillow pushes the head into a *Quirky Sideways* or *Tilted Head*. Keep the head level.

- Travel neck pillows make a good alternative if they fit comfortably under the neck and don't push on the skull.
- A simple, firm mattress often supports the skeletal structure more than one with all the "bells and whistles."
- Sleeping on a cot, couch, recliner, or hammock is not recommended, nor is a waterbed. *(Are they still around?)*

RECOVERY-BASED SOFT TISSUE THERAPY HABITS

Massage Habit

There's a high probability that the molding stretches will make your muscles achy, tight, and sore, especially in the beginning. It's entirely possible that the discomfort may not let up, and it could get fairly intense. That's when you will need to help your soft tissue recover so you can keep moving toward your Reverse Strategy goals. Just to be clear, the soft tissue discomfort will eventually subside. However, seeking the assistance of a Massage Therapist or coaxing your *significant other's* massaging hands can help make that happen faster.

When patients attended *The Good Back Habits Class*, we encouraged them to bring a partner. Our instructor, Lilly, showed the participants how to massage each other using a **massage chair** and expressed her belief that **every family should own one**. Lilly explained how muscle fibers are strained during the molding process, which makes them irritable, causes them to spasm, and painful knots (trapped lactic acid) develop. Then, she taught the class how to locate and treat them. Here is a shortened version of her *Press-Release-Massage-Method*. These home instructions are for a partner willing to help your muscles recover, or you can use this awesome technique on them.

Press—Release—Massage—Method

DISCOVER A–> Knot by using your thumb and deeply stroking along a muscle belly, muscle-tendon junction, and around a joint until you locate a painful "spot." You will find plenty of knots around the shoulder blades, hip joints, and forearms.

DEEPLY PRESS–> Down on the "spot" for 5 seconds. Release the pressure, then massage the area. Repeat 2-3 times more, (this may be very painful). If the correct "spot" was pressed, your subject should feel immediate improvement.

If you don't have a partner willing to press, release, and massage you, you will benefit greatly from seeking the care of a Massage Therapist. Massage isn't just for pampering oneself; it can help your achy and tight soft tissue recover from the constant push and pull of the molding stretches. This "soft tissue therapy habit" recommends seeing a Massage Therapist twice a month in year one.

RECOVERY-BASED FOOT THERAPY HABITS

Orthotics Habit

The goal of *The Bad Back To Good Back Method* is to restore stability (balance) to your skeletal structure. Along the way, all your joints should automatically function better. However, if running, golfing, hiking, or another activity still bothers your hips, knees, and/or feet, you may want to consider inserting orthotics into your footwear.

Here's the reason: there are 26 bones, 33 joints, and over 100 ligaments, tendons, and muscles that allow you to get your 4,000 steps in each day. The foot is a mechanical wonder, and it operates best when "the load" (body weight) it must carry is evenly distributed along the entire length of the foot.

Here's the problem: your Bad Back Type and its faulty skeletal parts have already altered "the load" on your weight-bearing joints, and your feet have been affected **more so** because they are the **last… joints… in… line** (it's just physics). When certain areas of the foot receive more stress, the foot joints will eventually succumb. That's why the feet will toe in or out, supinate or pronate, develop *fallen arches, hammertoes, heel spurs,* and any of the conditions listed below. Don't blame your feet; blame it on the joints **above** your feet (ankles, knees, hips, pelvis), and understand that whatever foot condition "ails you" is the result of your skeletal structure's **imbalances**. Check the soles of your shoes for wear and tear; that's where the foot is being stressed.

With the help of an orthotic, you can "restore balance" (stability) to your feet, which will help "restore balance" (stability) to your knee joints and all 5 pelvic joints. Then, "restoring balance" (stability) to your skeletal structure becomes a SNAP… and that is why I recommend wearing shoe orthotics as a Foot Therapy Habit.

When a Bad Back is on its way to becoming a Good Back, mechanically based hip, knee, and foot problems are going to improve anyway. If that's enough for you, good, that's the intention. However, if you want faster results and maybe resolution, obtain a pair of custom-made orthotics (see our website for this recommendation). Put them in every shoe, and wear them all… the… time because maintaining a Good Back takes a good amount of effort, but wearing an orthotic does not.

Supportive Footwear Habits

Whether or not you have hip, knee, ankle, or foot problems, you will need to be mindful of the shoes you wear. Not every shoe is going to be good for *The Good Back Type*, and some shoes could be downright bad. Choose your footwear wisely, and you will support the center alignment of your pelvis. Choose unwisely, and you'll likely push the pelvis out of alignment.

- Shoes with a "raised heel" force the body to lean forward so body weight falls onto the balls and toes of the feet. To negate the effects of wearing heels (even sneakers can have a wedge-type heel), try to remember to "stand at attention" whenever possible.

- Flat shoes (like penny loafers) are recommended.
- If you are not using orthotics, wear flat shoes with arch supports.
- Select a shoe with a material that supports and holds the foot in place. Flimsy material and most slippers allow the foot to "roam freely," which can create or worsen mechanically based foot problems.
- Enclosed shoes are more supportive than open-back sandal styles, and flip-flops (for the same reason as above).
- Shoes with a "pitched footbed" force the body to lean backward, so body weight falls onto the heels. That's the part of the foot that should "bear more load," so this type of shoe makes standing tall, straight, and proud with your head held high a—little—easier.
- Rocker-style shoes with an upward-angled footbed and flat heel (NOT a rocker heel) are the best choice for footwear.

A Pitched Footbed

It was a beautiful day when we spontaneously headed for the Adirondack Mountains. The next day, I anxiously dressed for a hike, but my shoe bag was nowhere to be found… *ugh!* I slipped my Keds® back on, grabbed coffee, and took the short walk to the local shop. They had everything for the outdoor enthusiast. With the attendant's guidance, I bought an unfamiliar brand of **very comfortable** hiking sneakers with this key selling point: "a pitched footbed."

When I put those shoes on, I knew exactly **why** they were a "hot-ticket item" for the shop. The toe box of this trail running shoe gradually, ever-so-slightly, angled upward, making it easier to stand upright. I'm telling you, not only were my feet happy, but I was instantly energized as I strolled down the sidewalk in this new-to-me shoe style, and I couldn't wait to share the news. See our website for this recommendation.

RECOVERY-BASED BACKBONE THERAPY HABITS

Adjustment Habit

The intention behind the Reverse Strategies is to push your faulty parts into their natural alignment. To accomplish this, you will lay over your orthopedic devices daily so they can "gently push" your muscles, ligaments, and joints. If your soft tissue doesn't mind being stretched and your bones move easily, reversing your Bad Back Type **should... be... a... cinch**. On the other hand, if your soft tissue is stiff and your joints are jammed or stuck, molding may be more uncomfortable than you can tolerate. This may make you feel like you aren't making any progress, and you might be right, but if you are thinking about throwing in the towel, wait just a minute... there's a **small detail** that I intentionally left out until now.

Soft tissue and joints that don't want to budge WILL NOT move with the "gentle push" of an orthopedic device. They need more force; they need the *adjustment*. I've given thousands of *adjustments* to patients ranging from tiny babies to the elderly. Nothing has been more rewarding than pushing, pulling, and twisting their backbone joints or—any of their skeletal joints—to help them feel and function better. Backbone Practitioners worldwide offer various methods and techniques for Backbone Therapy, but it's the *adjustment* that offers the best results. The *adjustment* is so effective that when it's coupled with the Reverse Strategies, it's like stepping on the gas pedal; your journey to *The Good Back Type* will be much—much faster.

The *adjustment* is a quick, forceful push, pull, or twist on backbone joints—or any skeletal joint. It's designed to break through soft tissue fibers to loosen the joints so they are primed and ready to be molded. Getting *adjusted* WILL hasten your pace as you take your Bad Back and make it a Good Back. In some cases, a single *adjustment* is good enough, but most of the time, it takes more than one. Blame it on scar tissue.

Scar tissue is the body's natural repair response to a wound or injury, like a cut in the skin, a strained muscle, or a sprained tendon or ligament. To repair damaged tissue, heavy-duty fibers are laid down in a crisscrossed pattern like this, XXX, to make the "new" skin, muscle, tendon, or ligament much tougher and far less stretchy. (*Ever chew on a piece of meat that wouldn't break down in your mouth, so you had to spit it out?* That was scar tissue.) *How does scar tissue affect the backbone?* Scar tissue is the reason ligaments thicken and stiffen, and the joints they hold together don't easily loosen. Scar tissue is why two, twelve, or twenty *adjustments* might be necessary to break through the soft tissue and free up the joints so they can be molded straight or into a curve.

The Pushing Adjustment

When a practitioner PUSHES on backbone joints—or any skeletal joint—the intention is to improve the "range of motion" to help jammed or stuck joints *move freely* and compressed nerves "obtain relief." The **biggest benefit** of the *pushing adjustment* is that bones can be pushed toward their Vertically Straight and Curvy Alignment. I'm a BIG FAN of this type of force because *pushing* allows joints to slide along their surface, which "respects and protects" the joint surface and backbone discs.

A Hot Mess

"Thursday morning, I drove to visit a friend four hundred miles away. The day after I arrived, I could feel a tightness at the base of my neck and between my shoulder blades that I could definitely blame on driving with my arms extended for six-and-a-half hours straight! I stretched like crazy, self-massaged the area, hydrated, and rested. Still, Friday's tightness turned to stiffness on Saturday, and a nice headache was developing at the base of my skull.

I was a hot mess when I returned home for Mother's Day activities, and several family members asked if I was tired because I looked haggard (I felt like that, too). On Monday, we golfed despite my headache and inability to turn my head. Later in the afternoon, three other symptoms appeared:

my cognition was compromised, I felt feverish, and my Right ear began to pulsate. I didn't join the family for dinner. When Tuesday arrived, I awoke with an earache.

I had finally reached the end of my rope! In front of the bathroom mirror, I stood as naturally as possible with my eyes closed. The Mirror-Mirror-Method Dr. Faith taught us really does work because half a minute later, when I opened my eyes, the mirror confirmed what I had felt; my chin was way off center!

Thankfully, Dr. Faith was available, and when I did the Skeletal Dance for her, she confirmed my Quirky Sideways Head. I laid my body sideways on the adjusting table and felt her familiar hand placed on my Atlas. She pushed quickly and forcefully a few times until we both felt the "clunk" of the joint movement. I felt it almost immediately but stood up so she could see if there was improvement. Yes, her mission was accomplished, and my head sat firmly in the center of my body. With renewed energy, my ear and neck issues completely gone (despite having felt like a train wreck just minutes before my adjustment), I grabbed my coat, and off to the grocery store, I flew. Dr. Faith has magical hands!"

The pushing adjustment isn't magic; it's just physics. Misaligned joints are pushed toward their natural alignment. That's it. By evaluating whether a faulty part has shifted sideways, twisted, or tilted, the practitioner can ***push it back*** (it's simple and quite effective).

The Pulling Adjustment

When a practitioner PULLS on backbone joints—or any skeletal joint—the intention is to improve the "range of motion." Adjusting joints by *pulling* them allows jammed or stuck joints to "reposition themselves" so they can *move freely,* and compressed nerves can "obtain relief." *The pulling adjustment* DOES NOT move bones toward their Vertically Straight or Curvy Alignment; however, *pulling* joints apart "respects and protects" the joint surface and backbone discs.

I'm a BIG FAN of *pulling* extremity joints (shoulders and hips, elbows, hands, fingers, knees, ankles, feet, and toes), which respond extremely well to this type of force, especially weight-bearing joints. For example, if you've ever had a painful knee or ankle joint that wouldn't allow you to put weight on it for almost no apparent reason, it was probably **jammed**, and the nerves compressed. If that joint was *pulled* apart, it could "reposition itself" to *move freely* again. Feeling and functioning much better, you would swear a miracle just occurred.

Bird Box

We were sitting by the fireplace when she flew **into** our sliding glass door so violently that Chief (our dog), Leo (our cat), and I bolted like lightning to the wreckage. With just a splash of red on her wings and an unmistakable crown and beak, I knew she was a female cardinal. This event was not unusual as the bird feeder is only thirty feet away from our deck, which makes the thud, remnants of feathers on the glass, and a bird gasping for air quite a sight.

I quickly ran to get the "bird box" stowed away in a nearby closet, then opened the door to pick her up. As I wrapped the dry washcloth around her head and body, she squawked loudly, so I softly reassured her that she would be all right. My Left hand held her body, and fingertips from my Right hand loosely gripped her cloth-wrapped head. With a firm tug, I pulled her skull once, twice with more force, and three times total. *There, I affirmed to myself, I'm sure one of those tugs separated her skull from her Atlas.*

The bird would surely have died like many before her if I hadn't rescued her. *Why?* Because their head slammed into the glass door with such force, it compressed their skull into their neck bones to create neurological pressure. They'd lay there for hours until their Life Force diminished, but some die instantly. Thankfully, I was home that day.

After her *adjustment*, I placed the bird in the box wrapped in the cloth, closed the lid, and said a prayer. Three hours later, when I opened the top just a smidge, she flew out so fast that she almost knocked me over. It was a great feeling to know that she would reunite with her partner and live to tell him about her adventure. Pulling joints decompresses them and relieves nerve pressure, and sometimes, it can be lifesaving.

The Twisting Adjustment

When a practitioner TWISTS backbone joints—or any skeletal joint—the intention is to improve the "range of motion" to help jammed or stuck joints *move freely* and compressed nerves "obtain relief." Twisting joints DOES NOT move bones toward their Vertically Straight or Curvy Alignment (unless it's to correct a *Quirky Twisted Head*).

I'm **NOT** a fan of this type of force (especially used long-term) because *twisting* causes friction on the joint surfaces (similar to opening a child-proof bottle cap), which wears them down, promotes arthritis, and may damage the discs wedged between the movable backbones.

AL's Story

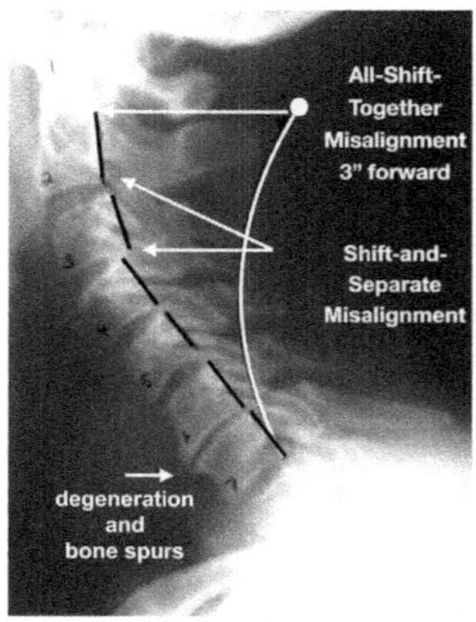

AL came to my office because he couldn't turn his head to back his car out of the driveway, and his Backbone Practitioner of fifty years had passed away. *WOW,* was my response, but it was also my reaction as we looked at his X-rays. AL's neck bones were degenerated and shifted forward about 3 inches! It was apparent that AL's exaggerated *Bowling Ball Head* had been *twisted* for 50 years… and… it goes without saying… adjusting the neck by *twisting* it DOES NOT stop the bones from shifting forward, but it DOES wear them down. To return AL's head to its natural alignment, he used the *Reverse Bowling Ball Head Strategy,* and by concentrating on that goal for a year, AL could back out of his driveway again.

Leo's Crooked—Tipped Tail

I can't resist telling this story about my cat's tail, which is crooked at the tip as if it got caught in a closing door. It's at a 90° angle. Leo was a feral cat when I discovered him living under my neighbor's house. After befriending him for months, I mustered the courage to trap him in my garage and eventually brought him inside my home for the long journey of domestication.

When Leo finally allowed me to touch the tip of his tail comfortably, seven months had passed, and curiosity was getting the best of me. One day, as he lay snuggled in my arms, I gently dragged my fingers to the end of his tail to "feel the spot." Indeed, there was a bend between two of his tiny tail bones. I clenched the tip, stretched it out, then gave a tiny but forceful tug once, twice, and with increasing force, a third time. I knew his tail bones wouldn't straighten out, not this time or any number of times I pulled on those joints, but I continued day after day for a week or so until my husband caught me. Obviously, I had to disclose my intentions by explaining that it was my little experiment.

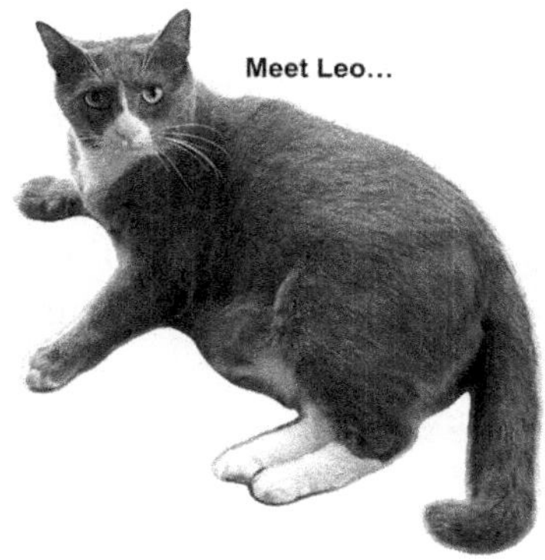

Me: *Many people think they can correct their backbone misalignments by getting adjusted. It's foolishness, just like my attempt to straighten Leo's crooked-tipped tail.*

John: *What would it take to straighten his tail?*

Me: *Well, I'd have to adjust the crooked part regularly, then bend it in the opposite direction from its current crooked position and hold it there for 20 minutes every day for a year and another year to cure.*

John looked at me with an expression I'll never forget: a cocked head coupled with rolled eyes!

When backbone joints—or any skeletal joints—are *pushed, pulled, or twisted* so that joint motion and/or joint alignment has improved, it's ONLY TEMPORARY. This means that joints will settle back into their old spot**... ugh...** nerve pressure/irritation will return**... double ugh...** and Bad Back Signs and *Quirky's* remain**... triple ugh!** Getting an adjustment ensures joints can *move freely,* but it DOES NOT guarantee they will **stay** where the adjustment moved them. The only way to ensure the bones stay in place is to mold them 20 minutes daily for a year and another year to *cure.*

Self Adjusting Is A Bad Habit

Self-adjusters **never** came to see me of their own accord; they were SENT to me by parents and spouses. They were mostly teenagers and married men who would show up at my office, insisting they didn't need me to *crack their joints* because they **did it** themselves.

Self-adjusters *crack their joints* to relieve built-up nerve pressure. The nerve endings (mechanoreceptors) within a joint capsule can only take so much pressure before they get irritable. This irritation causes the afflicted person to get very uncomfortable, and the only way to relieve the pressure is for them to move their joint. Most ***twist*** the joints. Because joints aren't moved toward their Vertically Straight or Curvy Alignment, they settle back into their "old spot," and nerve pressure returns.

When someone *cracks* their neck, it looks unpleasant and sounds horrifying, but that's only part of the problem. That person is compelled to *crack their joints* again and again because joint pressure is always present with *Bowling Ball Head,* for example. If misaligned bones were shifted back to their natural alignment, the "afflicted" wouldn't have to *crack* their neck bones repeatedly (which negatively affects joint surfaces and discs).

How did I handle these self-adjusters? I asked them to commit to "our method" for three solid months, promising them that the "urge to crack their joints" would be greatly diminished or completely gone. Written testimonials expressed happiness and surprise at their results. If you know someone who obsessively *cracks their joints,* do them a favor and recommend this book because *self—adjusting is a bad habit.*

A Force Got You Here A Force Must Take You Back

You developed a Bad Back Type with the help of a quick force accident or gravity's slow force. Now, another force must take you to *The Good Back Type.* If the orthopedic devices you are using are enough force to get the job done, **good**, that's the intention! However, if you want faster results, seek the quick force *adjustment* of a Backbone Practitioner, or choose a practitioner trained in *The Bad Back To Good Back Method* for lightning-fast results! This Good Back Habit recommends incorporating Backbone Therapy 1-4x/month in year one for an accelerated journey to *The Good Back Club.*

STEP 10: PROVE YOUR BAD BACK IS NOW A GOOD BACK

My Favorite Patient

One morning, I was at my computer writing this book when I got a call from my husband, John.

John: *Honey… I'm at Josh's shop, and a moment ago, I was standing behind the customer counter eating a bowl of granola. I bent slightly to take a mouthful, and suddenly, I felt like someone had stabbed me in the back. The pain grabbed me so fast that I almost lost my balance. Slowly, I made my way to a nearby chair, but I'm not quite sure how I did. I didn't lift anything this morning other than a propane cylinder, but that didn't seem to bother me. That wouldn't have caused this, right? I'm just trying to figure this whole thing out and work through it. Right now, I can't move from this chair and feel somewhat helpless. Do you think a muscle relaxant or aspirin would help? It feels like the same issue when I tweaked my back a few summers ago, but this time, there's a bit of shooting pain. Hello...?*

Me: *Yes, dear, sorry about my silence; I'm at my computer writing this down.*

John: *Oh, great… I'm not really sure why I called you, and there's nothing you can do, but I'm struggling to understand why this happened.*

This scenario is probably no different from any other professional who attempts to "assist" their friends and family. Let me explain my frustration… I have an open-door policy for giving *adjustments*, but they only come when their back problems get pretty bad. When I give recommendations like keeping up with their molding strategies, they usually don't comply. The latter was the case with John, and this was my response.

Me: *Okay, you want my opinion? Your first injury occurred when you were out on the boat ten years ago; five years ago, when you took the tree down,* *you re-injured yourself. Now, you are stuck at the shop, unable to get out of the chair, and you don't know WHAT caused this??? Here's what I know... After each episode, I adjusted you, and you molded your low-back until you felt better. Thinking your back was FIXED, you stopped molding. When you stopped molding, it was only a matter of time before your faulty parts shifted back into their old pattern: The Stoop.*

If you don't mold, even a little, you will re-injure those parts again and again because they're weak and vulnerable. Honestly, the strategies don't take any time out of your day because you're molding in bed as you fall asleep. If you stayed committed to molding a couple of times a week, you wouldn't be wondering how to get out of that chair. Today's episode is the backbone's fault, but it's really YOUR fault! Come on, dear, you know better.

There was silence for a few seconds.

John: *Okay, that's kinda what I thought you'd say; I'll figure this out. Bye.*

John hung up the phone, and half of my heart was sad that he'd have to go through the repair process AGAIN, but the other half of me was mad because the last time he re-injured himself, it took him twenty-seven days to recover!

Let John's **victim of re-injury** be a lesson. At some point along your "bad to good" journey, you will realize you feel good. Your pain will be gone, and molding might seem unnecessary. DO... NOT...STOP... MOLDING. Feeling good is wonderful, but don't let gravity pull you back into your *old pattern*. Review the strategy phases below to help you **avoid** falling *victim to re-injury.*

REVERSE STRATEGY MOLDING PHASES

These molding phases are a general "timeline guide" designed to help you navigate the molding process. They are divided into three periods: **Holding**, **Training**, and **Curing**. Each phase corresponds to the soft tissue and joint changes that are expected to occur during that time.

Holding Phase

This is the **hold that molding stretch** phase (Step 8, Rule #4). Your goal during this period is to push or pull the faulty parts into a molding stretch until you can easily and comfortably hold EACH Reverse Strategy for ALL 20 minutes straight. Some strategies are bound to be more challenging than others; don't panic, just **don't... give... up.** Mold every day, multiple times per day (if necessary) to reach the 20-minute mark, then follow the Training Phase.

Training Phase

The goal of this phase is to TRAIN the faulty parts to **stay in place.** You will accomplish this task by molding for one year. As you begin this 12-month countdown, you may reduce EACH Reverse Strategy to 3x per week (Step 8, Rule #11). Additionally, during this period, you will steadily increase the push to further challenge your faulty parts (Step 8, Rule #7). This means UPSIZE all your devices (if possible) during this molding year. At the 12-month mark, **validate** that your Bad Back is a Good Back (see below). For those reversing *Quirky's*, the recommendation is to mold until they resolve. Use the Skeletal Dance Mirror-Mirror Method to confirm (Step 6).

Curing Phase

This phase is reserved for those who have already trained their faulty parts for one solid year. The goal for this phase is to ensure the faulty parts CURE, **maintain placement**, so they don't shift back into their old pattern. This means you may "lighten up" on EACH Reverse Strategy to 2x per week for another 12 months (or indefinitely). Additionally, during this phase, it is recommended to UPSIZE your device sizes (if possible).

The above phases helped our patients better understand the entire molding process. Although helpful, most could gauge when they were ready to move from one phase to the next (some took their time, and others moved right along). With only this book as your guide, you'll decide how to proceed. I HAVE FAITH IN YOU.

VALIDATE YOUR BAD BACK IS GOOD AND JOIN THE CLUB

During my clinic days, we **validated** our patients' progress by comparing their *before and after* Structural Evaluations and X-rays. It was their moment of truth.

Did the time and effort they put into their treatment program pay off? Did their backbone actually undergo structural changes? Do they naturally stand in *The Good Back Type*?

This is your **moment of truth**. If you've spent sufficient time restoring your backbone curves and straightening the bent parts, it will be stronger, more stable, and springy. If you can NATURALLY stand in *The Good Back Type,* you are validating that **all... your... hard... work** has paid off.

Validation should follow the completion of the *Training Phase*. The best way to validate whether or not you can stand naturally in *The Good Back Type* is to **compare** your *before and after* pictures. Use your initial (side view) Structural Evaluation picture for your *before,* and follow the instructions below to take another picture for your *after*.

- Refer to Step 6, Actions #1–#5
- Wear similar clothes.
- Evaluate in the same place.
- Have the same **observer** take your picture.
- Use the same Evaluation Chart (obtained from our website).

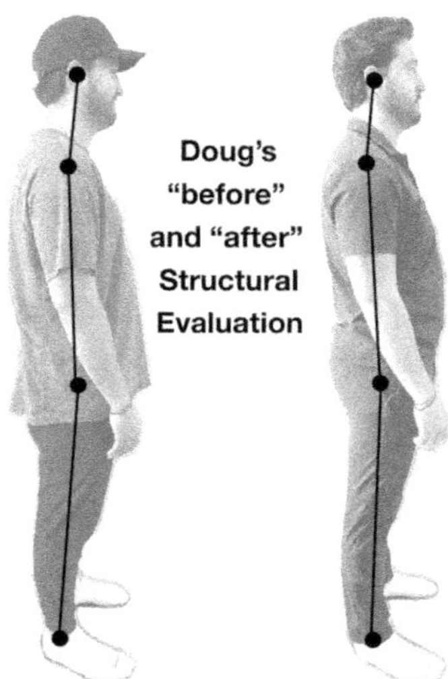

(Image 10A)

Comparing your *before and after* pictures, *can you say your Bad Back is now a Good Back?* Some people make small changes, like Doug, who applied "our method" for only a few weeks

(Step 6, Doug's Story), while others who mold for 12 months straight make huge changes.

Regardless of your improvements, congratulations, and allow me to applaud your membership into *The Good Back Club.* Send me your *before and after* pictures, and we will post you on our club webpage.

Happy When You Feel Good

One morning, a new patient questioned our front desk assistant as he returned his intake form. *"Why are the people here so happy? I've never seen a doctor's office filled with laughter; nobody acts like they're in pain. Do they have any back problems?"*

Sarah smiled and responded, *"At one time, these people were in lots of pain, but their pain is usually gone within a month. Most of these patients choose a treatment program that restores stability to their backbone, so they have regularly scheduled office visits. You'll learn more about this when you speak with Dr. Faith, but I can tell you one thing: The Good Back Method makes people feel good, and that's why they are happy."*

Lottie's Story

The first thing Lottie said as she made her way through our office door was, *"I want you to know I hardly go anywhere, but my nagging neighbor brought me to your talk, and I'm so glad I went."* **See Step 5, image 5B**. Remember, Lottie was the lady from the Senior Center who turned out to be a genuinely kind woman in her mid-seventies, plagued with a problem from her waist down. Born in the mid-thirties, she contracted the Polio Virus when she was fifteen (at the height of the polio pandemic). Hospitalized in a sanitarium for nearly a year, she sadly stated, *"I was never the same physically, mentally, or socially."*

Lottie's lower body was affected mainly by the damaged motor nerves, and as she aged, her weakened legs wouldn't allow her to stand too long or walk too far. Then, at age sixty-two, Lottie's pelvic area developed numbness. She said, *"I can't even feel myself poop, and when I walk, it feels as if I'm in quicksand up to my belly button."* With a loss of sensation, Lottie's lower extremities were always cold, which prompted her to lay a heating pad over her legs during the day, set her electric blanket on high at night, and wear socks to bed.

Lottie's condition was known as *Post Polio Syndrome*, but in my eyes, she had *Boobs Meet Belly* in an advanced stage. Lottie began her Reverse Strategies with enthusiasm, molding daily, and when she no longer needed to wear socks to bed, we ALL felt hopeful. Yet, it was her attitude that was truly inspiring. *"It doesn't matter what God gives you—make the effort to stand tall, straight, and proud with your head held high!"*

The Little Old Lady/Man Bad Back Type

Similarly, it doesn't matter what kind of condition your backbone is in… if you don't make an effort to reverse your *Bad Back Syndrome Type*, then your skeletal structure will degrade, degenerate, and eventually, it will become… *The Little Old Lady/Man Bad Back Type.*

This Bad Back Type will result when a person's skeletal structure succumbs to gravity's pull. Those already plagued with this "type" used to be full of life in their 40s and 50s, then in their 60s and 70s, they had to reduce their activity level due to physical limitations. In their 80s, their severe physical problems matched their severe health problems, and they blamed the *aging process* instead of the *downward slide* of their skeletal structure. As Rule 13 already warned, if you want to avoid this scenario, start reversing your "type" now and MOLD FOR LIFE because if you "let up" on staying upright, your structure... will let you down.

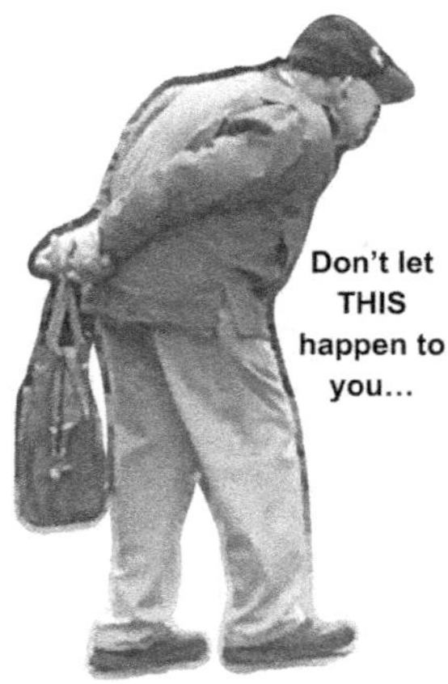

(Image 10B)

Consider this: Johnny's skeletal structure is made of a hard plastic material that will never change, but your flesh n' bones can be changed (with a fair amount of effort). Start taking care of your bony structure NOW so you don't end up looking like Johnny as you age… stuck in a hunched-over and sideways lean! See Johnny's Obituary, pages 16-17; sorry to disappoint, he's not real.

There Are NO Absolutes

This is my default statement regarding the condition of your skeletal structure and whether or not the material in this book can help improve it. My guidance may be the whole answer to your back problems or only a part of it. We are all unique individuals, and what works for one person may not work for another.

The Reverse Strategies in Step 7 should help restore the strength, stability, and springy-ness to your backbone; however, underlying "disorders" may prevent you from obtaining the results you desire. Do the best you can to identify and resolve your *Bad Back Syndrome Type* with the information given. If nothing else, you'll be preserving your skeletal structure from moving toward the grave (that I can assure you).

There are no guarantees that *The Bad Back To Good Back Method* will eliminate your back problems, but it can help you stand tall, straight, and proud with your head held high until the end of your days.

About the Author

Bad Back Syndrome causes back pain and many other problems involving muscles, nerves, joints, and discs. It's a condition that Dr. Faith Miller, a Backbone Practitioner of nearly 30 years, coined to help expel the mystery and complexity surrounding the age-old question, *"What's WRONG with my back?"*

Along the way, she discovered that people don't need complicated medical jargon—they **want** the truth. They **need** the truth explained in everyday language that they can understand and apply. That realization led to the development of the *Bad Back to Good Back Method* and ultimately her book, The Real Reason Your Back (still) Hurts.

With decades of experience, Dr. Faith has empowered patients to use her method to take care of their own back. Now, her new book helps the *do-it-yourselfer* discover the root cause of their back pain and problems (Bad Back Syndrome), learn how to reverse that condition, and experience lifelong relief.

This is unlike any other book you've ever read; entertaining, full of easy-to-grasp terminology, and a simple, step-by-step system that will have you scratching your head, wondering why nobody else is talking about this stuff, much less teaching it.

As an author, speaker, and coach, Dr. Faith's mission is to help people, just like you, FIX THEIR OWN BACK! She states, *"There is nothing more rewarding for me than to help YOU help yourself."*

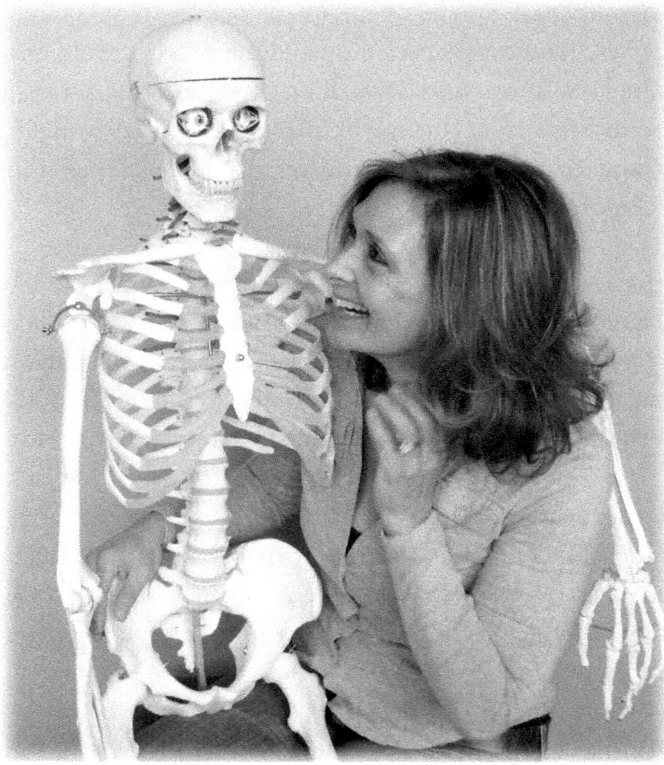

BAD BACK TO GOOD BACK

The Easiest, Most Effective Do-It-Yourself Method For Getting Rid Of Back Pain And Problems, Permanently!

www.ingramcontent.com/pod-product-compliance
Lightning Source LLC
Chambersburg PA
CBHW050527240926
51846CB00003B/724
* 9 7 8 1 9 6 1 7 8 1 8 4 9 *